A
COMPLETE
FITNESS
PROGRAM
FOR
PARTNERS

working out together

A
COMPLETE
FITNESS
PROGRAM
FOR
PARTNERS

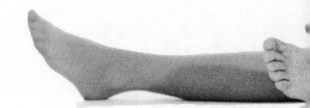

working out

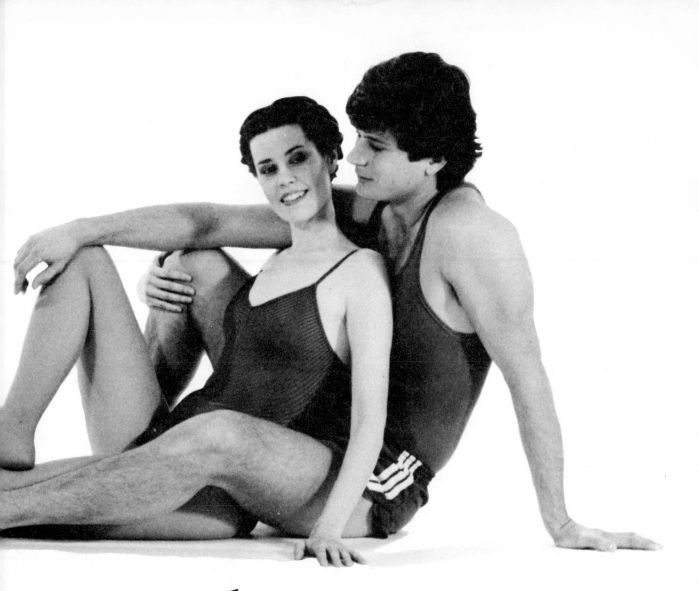

together

by CAROL GREGOR

Photographs by Pauline Augustine

BERKLEY BOOKS, NEW YORK

for Mom and Dad

WORKING OUT TOGETHER

A Berkley Book/published by arrangement with Lynn Sonberg Book Services

PRINTING HISTORY
Berkley trade paperback edition/April 1983

ISBN: 0-425-05878-6

acknowledgments

I want to thank my family—Harry, Chris, Alison, Florence, Arline— and friends—Brian, Robert, Elaine, Walter—not only for their en- couragement and support but for knowing when to leave me alone!

Special thanks to models Laura Hembree, Laurance Mont- gomery, Wendy Stuart, and Michael Harrison. Also to Sporting Woman and The Athlete's Foot in New York City for the use of their exercise clothes.

And my deepest gratitude and thanks to Lynn Sonberg for her invaluable counsel, patience, and time, without which I never could have written this book.

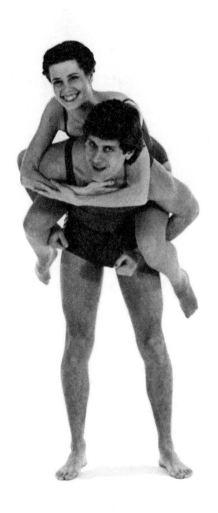

contents

1
why together? 1

2
getting started 4

3
building a better body: how the program works 8

4
the program 15

A. the warm-up	**16**
B. upper body exercises: arms, shoulders, chest, neck, and back	**31**
C. lower body exercises: midriff, waist, abdomen, buttocks, and hips	**67**
D. exercises for legs and feet	**94**
E. cardiovascular exercises	**121**
F. the cool-down	**144**

exercising alone 156

special cases: exercises for sports and problem spots 174

unwinding together 189

eating for fitness 199

keeping it all together 207

suggested reading 208
the program chart 211
sample exercise program 212
new american eating guide 214

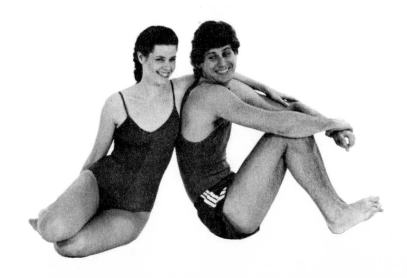

why together?

1

MARILYN AND JOHN have been married for over twenty years, but you'd never know it to look at them. They both seem so youthful, energetic, and vibrant, at ease with themselves and the world. Especially Marilyn. Slim and graceful, she's over forty but she looks at least ten years younger. When she and John leave their apartment building in the morning on their way to their jobs, they part with real reluctance, almost as if they were newlyweds.

For Marilyn, this sense of well-being is a comparatively recent development. Not so long ago, she and John were drifting apart. While John jogged and swam and played tennis regularly, Marilyn was getting virtually no exercise at all. Her former major activity—running after their two children—was a thing of the past; her days were now spent at an interesting but sedentary job. Like many people who don't exercise regularly, she tired easily and was often listless and irritable. Not to mention that her figure was spreading in all directions.

"Haven't you ever followed a regular exercise regimen?" I asked her.

"I never had to," she replied. "I was always too busy with the children. Now, I don't know where to start! And I hate the thought of exercising alone!"

"You don't have to," I told her. "You can exercise with John. I guarantee you he'd be delighted."

"But I'm so out of shape! I could never keep up with him," Marilyn protested.

This was true, but the problem was easily remedied with a special preconditioning program that raised Marilyn's fitness level. Once she felt more comfortable and in control of her body, she and John happily embarked on the total fitness program for couples, a unique eight-week learning experience that lays the groundwork for a lifetime of good health and fitness.

Why is this program so successful? Because it takes care of the *whole* body: 100 percent of you will be limbered, strengthened, and toned. It's a program for anyone and everyone, from age sixteen to sixty, whether married, dating, or just friends, a program that will bring physical and psychological rewards that no other exercise plan offers.

Working with a partner means that much of the boredom that exercising alone can bring is exchanged for an experience that is both companionable and fun. But even more important, you are not merely exercising together, you are exercising each other as well. Each exercise is specifically designed to utilize each partner's resistance and strength for the benefit of both. It's somewhat like working with a Nautilus machine or lifting weights, except that the person providing the resistance is getting the rewards of isometric exercise. Thus a total conditioning process is *always* going on. Not a moment, not a movement is wasted!

The *core* of the couples' program, however, is designed to free you from the harmful effects of stress while tuning your body to the peak of physical fitness. Stress is one of the major factors affecting our health today. Besides being implicated in the onset of various diseases, stress drains energy and vitality. Although there is no better tension release known than exercise, I'll also show you breathing and massage techniques geared to help you relax.

Now, I know it can be difficult to work up enthusiasm for a regular exercise program. If you feel any hesitation in the beginning, perhaps it will help to view your exercise sessions as a routine obligation, like brushing your teeth or combing your hair. But I guarantee you that any initial reluctance will be short lived: exercising regularly, as any fitness enthusiast will tell you, quickly becomes infectious, and doing it with a partner makes it even more so! It won't be long before you will both be looking forward to your workout sessions, nor will it be long before the increased energy and strength you feel give you a noticeably more attractive appearance and attitude. Looking good and feeling good is an unbeatable combination. The winning attitude that comes with good health is contagious. It can be yours in as few as eight weeks.

The time to start is now!

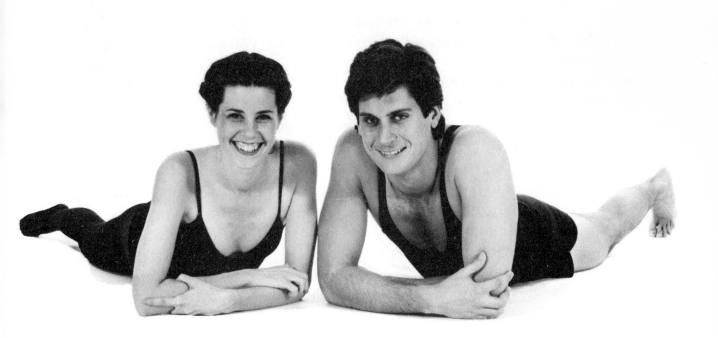

WHY TOGETHER?

getting started

2

LET'S SAY *you've* made the decision to begin. Congratulations! Now, how about your partner? Although he or she may understand the benefits of this program as well as you do, your partner might resist the idea of exercising with you. Why? One reason might be embarrassment. People are embarrassed about all kinds of things. Sometimes the closer they are to you, the more embarrassed they are. A friend might be easier to enlist in an exercise regimen than your spouse or lover. Perhaps your partner fears looking foolish or unattractive. Will that spare tire show? How about those heavy thighs? Or there might be more deeply seated psychological issues operating here, such as fear of failure or the need always to be the best.

Even if your partner's initial reaction isn't encouraging, don't give up. This program may be the best investment you ever make in your health and well-being *and* your relationship, so be persistent. Sit down and have a heart-to-heart talk. You may have some reservations as well. Admit them frankly, and tactfully encourage your partner to do the same. After all, the eventual benefits of the program far outweigh any of the possible drawbacks. It's a fantastic feeling to be really fit and full of energy, and there is no better method of achieving this than through exercise. And "being physical together" is a marvelous way to develop feelings of emotional closeness.

The most important thing is to get started. Though you may both feel self-conscious at first, that will soon pass. If you both openly discuss your feelings, any self-consciousness you have will pass even more quickly. In short order, you will be very much at home with your own—and each other's—bodies. You will feel invigorated, less tired, and much more "in touch" both physically and emotionally—the best possible kind of togetherness!

Where

You don't need a fully equipped gym or an area the size of a football field—just a space large enough for two bodies to lie down full length, allowing for one full arm's length behind the head and out to the sides. If you live in a warm climate and have a private outdoor area suitable for exercise, by all means use it and get the added bonus of fresh air and sunshine. Whether your space is indoors or outdoors, carpeted, bare floor, or grass, always use a small mat or towel under your bodies.

Privacy is essential. Close the door and take the telephone off the hook, and/or tell your family and friends to stay away during your exercise time.

If you are exercising inside, make sure you have proper ventilation. It's a good idea to air out the room about one hour before you start each session. During your winter sessions, keep the window open a crack. We are so used to overheated rooms that we have come to think that hot is good and any cool, fresh air that drifts in will cause colds. Just the opposite is true. We eliminate poisonous wastes from our systems as we breathe, exhaling the toxins and then refilling our lungs with clean, fresh air. Exercising in a poorly ventilated room means refilling your lungs with the toxins you have just gotten rid of.

A large mirror is desirable, though not necessary. If you have one, use it to watch how you work. Pretend you're watching someone else and observe yourselves with a critical eye. Check to see that your tummies are tight, your backs straight, and your shoulders relaxed. I'll give you more detailed instructions about what to look for in the exercise section itself.

When

It's your decision; pick whatever time suits your schedules best. Though there are no hard and fast rules, most couples choose early mornings or early evenings. If you're having your sessions at lunch time, there's no reason why you can't eat something light before beginning: a bowl of soup, a cup of yogurt, or a piece of fruit. It's usually better, however, to eat afterwards. Under no circumstances should you ever exercise after a heavy meal. At best, it will make you feel sluggish, and at worst ill!

Once you have worked out a schedule, stick with it. Be on time for your sessions. Don't arrive late or unprepared just because it is a personal rather than a business appointment. If an emergency arises, it should be easy enough for you to reschedule your workout session. Neither of you should cancel an exercise appointment, however, unless it is absolutely necessary, and then you should try to give the other at least twenty-four hours notice. Treat your commitment to the program with respect.

What to wear

Wear whatever you like, but remember, *comfort* is everything! T-shirts, shorts, leotards, bathing suits, jogging outfits—all are good choices. You shouldn't be aware of what you are wearing—remove all jewelry, belts, hair ornaments—and ladies, please, never, *never* wear a girdle while exercising. And unless the lack of support makes you uncomfortable, you should even remove your bra.

If your exercise area is cool during the winter, start your session wearing two layers of clothing. The layer next to the skin should be cotton, which allows perspiration to evaporate. A light sweater worn over the cotton layer will keep you warm. As soon as your exercises begin to make you warmer, remove the sweater. Wool is a good outer layer because even when it is wet with perspiration, it will not draw away your body heat. Wool leg warmers are excellent for keeping your leg muscles warm and limber. I'd advise you not to wear wool directly against your skin, since it can be itchy.

If your exercise area is warm enough, consider exercising naked.

Unclothed you are much more aware of your body's form, its strengths and vulnerabilities. You can actually see the effect of the exercise on specific muscle groups. Exercising together in the buff can be an exhilarating experience as well. But if either of you feels even the *slightest* bit uneasy or embarrassed about doing it, don't.

A word to the wise

As you progress with the program, the basic rule is to keep it fun. Although competing can be enjoyable, keep in mind that the program is not a contest. If you turn it into one, you'll miss out on its benefits. Remember, the program is a *shared* adventure toward excellence.

Having fun does not mean indulging in a lot of idle chatter. You should be relaxed and friendly during your sessions, but please be serious. Devote your time solely to doing the exercises; any talk should be about them. There is time to talk of other things later. Make your exercise time special and keep it that way!

Never forget that you are doing something really important for yourselves with a friend or a lover. Don't make light of it with acquaintances or, worse, treat it as a joke. Take it, and yourselves, seriously. This kind of physical contact with someone you are close to can be an extraordinary experience. You both have the privilege of getting to know another body as well as you know your own, and this familiarity with and trust in one another can develop into the sort of physical and emotional closeness you may never have experienced before. I can think of no better way to eliminate barriers and cement any relationship!

building a better body: how the program works

3

RECENTLY a friend of mine jokingly said while explaining his vigorous fitness regimen to me, "I don't care about my health; I just don't want to be fat!" Well, though said in jest, truer words have never been spoken!

For most of us the real motivation toward fitness is the desire to look great. What we're worried about is flabby thighs, drooping bottoms, thickening waists, or protruding abdomens. While the exercises that follow will definitely help you to develop and maintain a firm, sleek body, they are also designed to get you and keep you in the best possible health.

Without a regular fitness regimen, your muscles gradually lose their strength and your body loses its agility. Even while we are still in our twenties, if we do not engage in regular exercise our muscle tone, circulation, flexibility, and endurance can—and generally do—start going downhill.

Think back. Have you ever been too sick or too busy to get any exercise at all for several weeks? I bet that the first time you did anything physical again, you found that your body was stiff, weaker than usual, uncoordinated, perhaps even flabby. If you think about this situation in terms of *years* instead of weeks, you'll have a pretty good idea of how debilitating and destructive the lack of exercise can be.

Being weak and unfit can affect all areas of your life, personal *and* professional. Fatigue will overshadow even the simplest activity. This often becomes a vicious cycle: The less you do, the less energy you have, and thus the more lackluster and out of shape you become. The exciting news is that this kind of "aging" can quite literally be reversed. The body is a wonderfully responsive organism if you give it half a chance. No matter how out of shape you have let yourselves become, you can always restore your bodies to a healthier, firmer, more supple condition. Healthier people tend to be happier people—it's hard to be depressed when you're feeling so good and have the physical energy to pursue your heart's desire, whether it's an emotional commitment, a new product line at work, or a research project you've always wanted to undertake. This is nothing new; the ancients knew all this way back then. "*Mens sana in corpore sano*," they said. "A healthy mind in a healthy body."

What *is* new is that these days women as well as men are the happy beneficiaries of the realization that regular exercise is important to a happy and productive life. Once women were expected, even *encouraged*, to be frail. Being weak was considered the ultimate in femininity; having muscles was downright improper, and heaven help the woman who bested a man at any sport! Fortunately, women no longer need to repress their natural instincts toward excellence. Today, physical fitness is deemed as essential for women as it is for men. Both sexes are at their best when they are strong, glowing with health, and functioning at peak efficiency. And, perhaps not surprisingly, regular exercise has proved to be extremely useful in helping to eliminate problems that have consistently plagued women, such as low back pain (especially prevalent among pregnant women and new mothers), fatigue, depression, menstrual problems, and overweight.

As you embark on your eight-week program to total fitness, consider this: Being at your peak both physically and mentally is something you owe yourselves. You can't give your best to others if you haven't first given it to yourselves.

Building endurance: how your muscles work

As your total body strength increases, so will your endurance. You'll find yourself being able to do more and more. Why? Because when you work out on a regular basis, your muscles' capacity to store and burn fuel is improved. The primary fuel used for exercise is *carbohydrates*, which the body stores in the muscles and liver in the form of *glycogen*. A secondary source of fuel is *fat*, which is stored in the muscles and under the skin. Also necessary for exercise is *protein*. Although it is not a source of immediate energy, it provides fuel after undergoing a chemical conversion and it helps the muscles and tissues to repair themselves. Another essential component is *potassium*, a mineral released from the muscle cells to help control heat buildup during exercise.

In order to burn fuel, muscles require oxygen. You will find that as your level of fitness improves, so does your bodies' ability to bring oxygen to your muscles via your bloodstreams. When glycogen is burned, it breaks down into a chemical called *pyruvate*. If there is enough oxygen available, pyruvate converts to *carbon dioxide*, which is then discharged through your pores and lungs. If, however, not enough oxygen is available to the muscles, pyruvate converts to *lactic acid* instead. Lactic acid buildup makes it increasingly difficult for your muscles to function. You begin to get tired, *very* tired. An extremely high level of lactic acid can even cause your muscles to cramp. That is why one of the most important favors you can do for yourselves, if you haven't done so already, is to learn to breathe deeply and rhythmically while exercising, so that your lungs draw in the maximum amount of oxygen possible.

Proper breathing is the key to effective exercise. Most people, given the chance, will hold their breath when exercising, particularly for the exertion phase of any exercise. In fact, exhaling for the exertion and inhaling for the release makes an exercise much more effective and permits the body to work with rather than against whatever force is at play.

Breathe through your nostrils, drawing the air through the back of your throat, comfortably filling your lungs. Concentrate on the back of your throat, not the bridge of your nose. Now exhale through your mouth; make a "whoosh" sound as you empty your lungs. Don't force either the inhale or the exhale; as you become more practiced, your lung capacity will gradually increase.

The way professional athletes and experienced fitness enthusiasts go about their endurance training is to continue an exercise session beyond the point that their muscles have used up their available supply of glycogen and have started burning fat. By frequently exercising past glycogen depletion and on to "the burn," in time you will build up the ability of your muscles to store glycogen. The more glycogen your muscles can store, the more endurance you'll have. Finally, frequent depletion of glycogen will eventually induce the muscles to burn fat *and* glycogen simultaneously. This is a much more efficient way to exercise than burning glycogen alone. It is toward this endurance level that you will be aiming.

Assessing your fitness level

Before undertaking the total fitness program, each of you should take this simple twelve-part fitness test to determine whether you need additional conditioning work before you begin.

1. Sit on a couch or on the floor with one leg tucked under you.

2. Reach an object two feet above your head by standing on tiptoe.

3. Stand with your feet together; without bending your knees, touch the floor with your hands.

4. Kneel and then sit back so your buttocks touch your heels, then lean forward and touch the ground in front of your knees with your forehead without raising your buttocks from your heels.

5. Sit cross-legged, with your feet tucked under you. Now get up without using your hands.

6. Balance on the toes of one foot for the count of 10; then a 10-count on the other foot.

7. Balance on your right leg, then bend to a flat-back position with your left leg extended out behind you. Now balance on the left leg and repeat.

8. Stand with your legs apart; bend forward to a flat-back position and bring your arms out to form a T. Your head should be up, eyes looking forward. Swiftly turn your trunk from side to side 20 times, alternately

touching the floor with your right, then your left hand, while the other hand (and arm) is pointing straight upward.

9. Stand straight; clasp your hands against the back of your head with your elbows out to the side. Keeping your back straight, bend your knees so weight is on toes. Straighten up. Now, raise your left knee and, twisting your torso, try to touch your knee with your right elbow. Repeat the exercise with your right knee and left elbow, starting from your original position. Do 10 times each side, as smoothly as possible.

10. Standing with your legs apart, clasp your hands together and stretch your arms straight above your head. Bend forward and rapidly bring your arms down between your legs, then straighten up again. Do this 20 times.

11. Sit with your knees bent and feet firmly on the floor. Tilt your chin in toward your chest and stretch your arms forward. Slowly roll back along the full length of your spine until you are flat on your back. Next, stretch your arms behind your head, then swing them gently forward and slowly roll back up to your original position. Do this with perfect control 3 times.

12. Lie on your back, arms stretched out to form a T. Pull your knees in toward your chest, then lower them to the floor on your right side. Then bring them over onto the left side. Do this 3 times while keeping your shoulders pressed to the floor.

If you can successfully do eight or more of these exercises, you are ready to start the program. (And congratulations on being in better condition than most people!) Anything less than eight means you need to devote some time to shaping up before you begin. Work with the "Exercising Alone" program in chapter 5 for two weeks, then take this test again. If there is a great disparity between your partner's and your fitness levels and only one of you needs to do additional work, there's no reason why you both can't start on the "Exercising Alone" program together. Then, when you're both ready, you can move on to the couples' program.

Note: No exercise program should be started without a complete physical and a clean bill of health from your doctor. For those of you with *any* history of pain—in the back, knees, elbows, shoulders, wherever—consulting your doctor is especially crucial since only he or she can determine the exact cause of the pain and whether it is safe for you to undertake an exercise program.

Before you start

In order to get the full benefit of the program, you should be relaxed enough to concentrate totally on what you are doing. If there's a possibility you may be too tense to get the most out of the program, precede your workout with the relaxation exercises found in chapter 7, "Unwinding Together." If you find these exercises difficult, chances are you should be spending extra time on them. Make them a regular part of each session.

If the relaxation exercises prove painful, it may be that you have many "tension blocks"—your muscles can't "let go." If this is the case and if you have gotten a clean bill of health from your doctor and you know, therefore, that the pain is not your body telling you that something is wrong, slowly and gently work through the pain. *Never* force yourself. Eventually the exercises will get increasingly easier as your muscles begin to relax. It's important to learn how to convert your tension energy into positive energy, since this will greatly enhance your ability to exercise properly. Being fully in touch mentally with your body movements as you do the exercises is an absolute must.

All of the exercises in the eight-week program have been carefully designed and arranged in a particular sequence so that you will receive the maximum benefit from each workout. It's essential that you follow the program exactly as designed. For your convenience, we have set up a chart (The Program, page 211) that tells you exactly what is required on each day. On the second day of the second week, for example, you will be doing the easy program, with the addition of cardiovascular segment E-1. To help you fully understand how the program works and how to use it, we have included a Sample Exercise Program (pages 212–213), which lists specific groups of exercises to do on specific days. You might want to follow this program until you are familiar enough with all the exercises to decide what sort of groupings work best for you, whether it be this sample program or your particular variation on it.

The program is divided into four segments, each lasting two weeks. Each week has three exercise sessions. Try to space these sessions with a rest day in between. Sessions on Monday, Wednesday, and Friday, for example, would be ideal. This isn't a hard and fast rule; obviously there will be times when you'll have no alternative to placing sessions back to back. Nonetheless, a rest day is desirable: it gives your muscles time to recover from the previous workout and also for any minor injuries to heal.

Having a rest day does not mean doing nothing! On your "day off" you might make it a point to walk, as fast and as far as possible, or to bypass elevators and climb the stairs instead. Rest day is also a perfect time to practice stretching exercises or to concentrate on additional relaxation techniques.

The exercises are classified according to level of difficulty: easy, medium, or hard ((E) , M , H). As you advance from one two-week segment to the next, you will also advance into the next area of difficulty. By the second half of the program (the third and fourth segments), you will be doing hard level exercises. If, during the fourth segment (the last two weeks), you are in such good shape that the exercises are not really challenging you, wear two-and-one-half-pound weights on your wrists and ankles during the sessions. (These weights are available in most sporting goods stores.)

Each exercise session is divided into five parts: A) warm-up exercises; B) upper body exercises, which concentrate on the muscles in the neck, shoulders, and arms; C) lower body exercises, which concentrate on the muscles in the midriff area, abdomen, buttocks, and hips; D) exercises for the legs, thighs, and feet; and F) cool-down exercises. There is also a cardiovascular exercise segment, E, to be added on day two of each week. It, too, has three successively more difficult sections, designated E-1, E-2, and E-3 on the program charts (within the Cardiovascular Exercises section of the book, these are designated (E) , M , and H , respectively).

The basic program is designed to be completed in thirty minutes, although you will probably need a little more time until you become familiar with the exercises. The cardiovascular segment will add approximately ten to twelve minutes to the session.

Good luck and good health!

the program

4

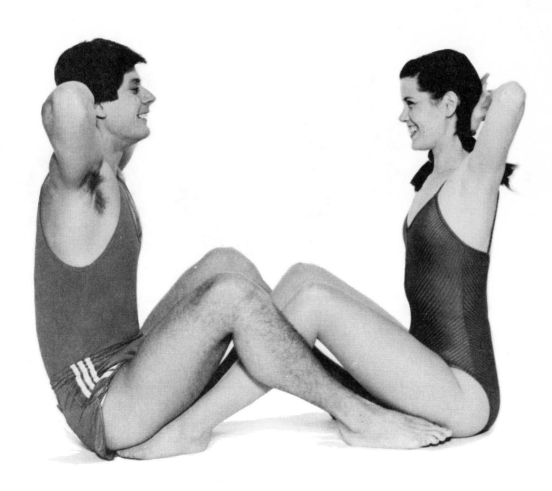

A. the warm-up

Roller Coaster　　Torso Twist

Shoulder Press　　Wraparound

Press and Twist　　Twist

Push and Pull　　Up-Down Seesaw

Side to Side　　Toe Tap

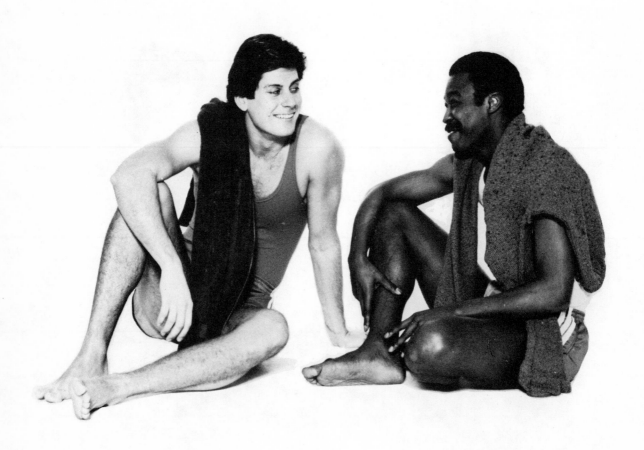

THE WARM-UP is one of the most important parts of your exercise session. Don't ever make the mistake of thinking you can skip it. Without it your bodies are no more prepared for serious exercise than you are prepared to go out on a winter day without overcoats!

During the warm-up, you take in more oxygen, which is absorbed by the blood, and increase the blood flow to your muscles. This oxygen-rich blood nourishes the muscles, making them more pliable. Once you are properly warmed-up, your bodies are protected against muscle strain and even more serious injuries such as muscle and ligament pulls or tears.

In this sequence of exercises, the major muscle groups come into play, starting with the muscles in your head and shoulders and continuing on down throughout your body to the legs. Your body's full range of motion is utilized: you are stretched from right to left, left to right, up and down, backward and forward.

Certain areas of the body are particularly susceptible to injury—the lower back, knees, elbows, and hips—so they need special attention. Follow the special precautions in the exercise segments to protect these vulnerable areas.

Like all the segments of this exercise program, the warm-up is designed to totally utilize the strengths and weaknesses of any couple by balancing flexibility with strength, endurance with fragility, so that the two of you together make a perfect, happy, and healthy whole.

ROLLER COASTER

BENEFITS This is a wonderful stretch for the whole body, particularly the chest and lower back. It is also good for developing coordination and grace.

THE EXERCISE Standing side by side, place one arm across each other's backs, palm on shoulder. Stand straight, keeping your feet a few inches apart.

Each of you stretch your free arm up and back, arching your backs. Lift up from your waists and reach back as far as you can, inhaling deeply. Now sweep forward in an arc, bending from the waist, and lower your hands to the floor. Exhale. Relax into the stretch and count to 3, breathing deeply. Then sweep forward and up once again. Repeat the sequence 6 times.

DOS AND DON'TS Keep your feet firmly on the floor, in a slightly turned out position. Don't rush; concentrate on achieving a smooth, flowing motion. If you cannot reach your partner's shoulder without throwing yourself off balance, place your hand wherever it's most comfortable.

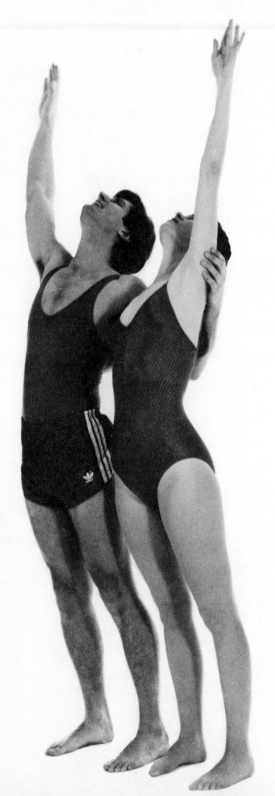

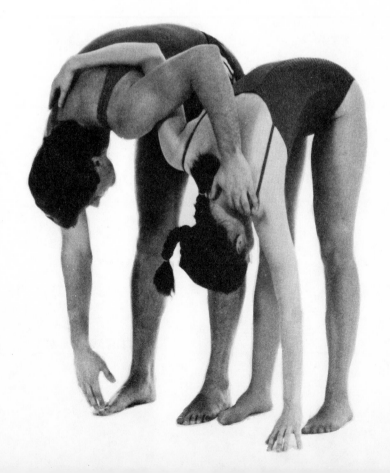

SHOULDER PRESS

BENEFITS This gently stretches the entire body, particularly the lower back and the backs of the legs.

THE EXERCISE Stand facing each other about two feet apart. Reach forward and place your hands on each other's shoulders and bend forward from the waist to the flat-back position.

Press your palms against each other's shoulders and bounce. Bounce as low as you can *without straining*. Do this 30 times, resting between each set of 10 bounces for about ten seconds. Breathe normally.

DOS AND DON'TS Don't let your stomach muscles droop; keep them contracted. Allow the lower back muscles to stretch in a smooth and gentle fashion. Keep your backs straight by tucking your buttocks under and holding your pelvises forward. Don't strain or force the motion.

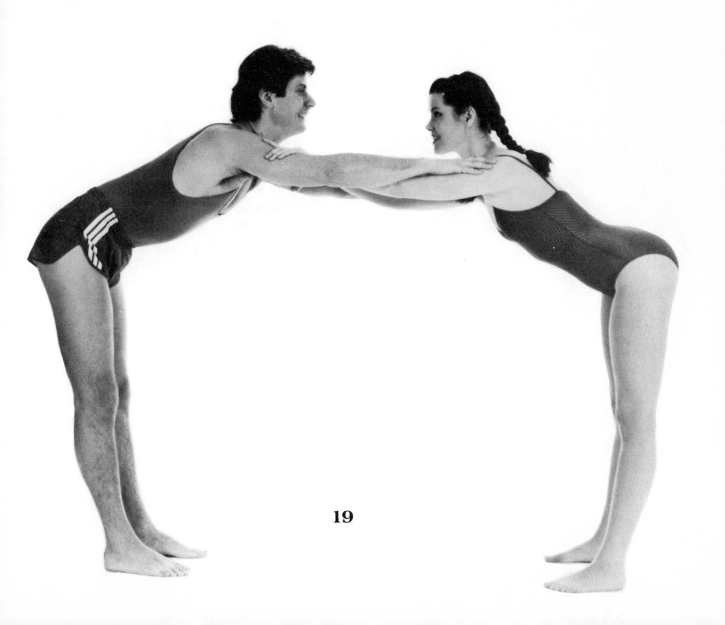

PRESS AND TWIST

BENEFITS This exercise benefits the lungs and general circulation, as well as increasing flexibility in the torso and taking off inches around the waist. It also stretches the lower back and legs.

THE EXERCISE Stand facing each other about two feet apart. Reach forward and place your hands over each other's shoulders. Bend forward from the waist to a flat-back position.

Press your palms on each other's shoulders and twist your torsos first to the right, then to the left. Do this set of twists 5 times, then return to the flat-back position and breathe deeply, exhaling for a count of 3, inhaling for a count of 3, then *holding* for a count of 3 while you tighten your abdomens. Repeat the breathing cycle.

Repeat the sequence for a total of 10 times with deep breathing cycle between each twist cycle.

DOS AND DON'TS Remember to breathe while twisting: inhale between twists, exhale as you twist. Keep your legs firmly placed but do not lock your knees. If you cannot reach your partner's shoulders, place your hands on his upper arms.

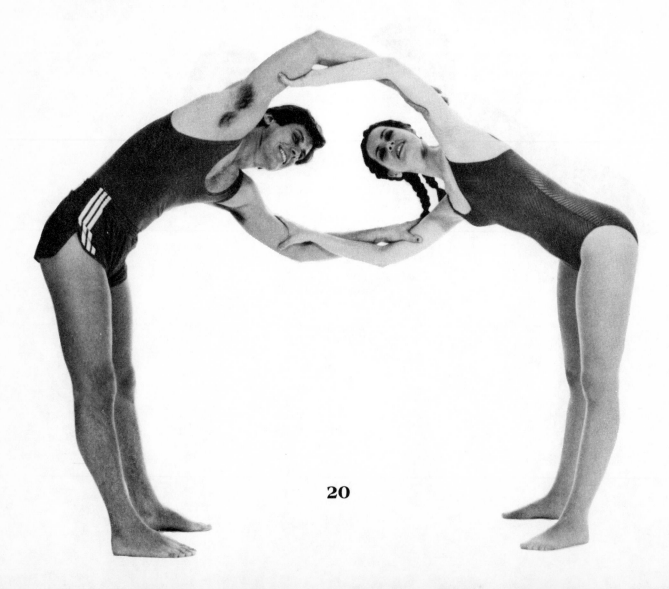

PUSH AND PULL

BENEFITS This is a wonderful exercise for the chest, upper back, and shoulder muscles. In addition, it will help make the entire spine flexible, take off inches around the waist, and strengthen the arms.

THE EXERCISE Sit facing each other with your legs crossed. Reach forward and take each other's wrists and raise your arms to shoulder level.

Push against each other's left hands while pulling on the right, twisting your upper bodies to the right and back. Then reverse, pushing right, pulling and twisting left. Repeat the sequence 30 times, stopping after each set of 10 to rest for a count of 10.

DOS AND DON'TS Twist back as far as you can, remembering to keep your elbows up. Remember to stay lifted through your chests, do not sag backward. Don't hold your breath during any part of this exercise.

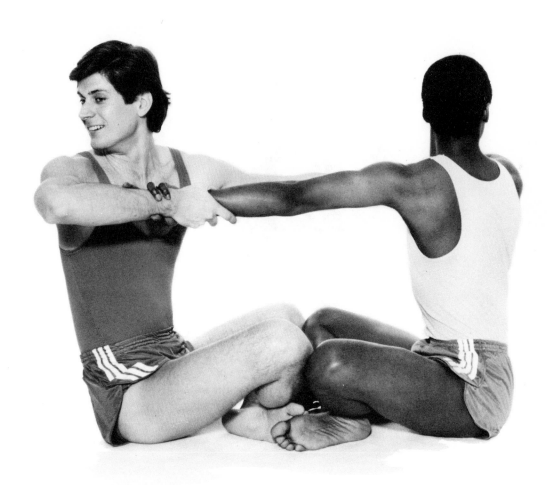

SIDE TO SIDE

BENEFITS This is an excellent stretch for the waist, hips, and inner thighs. It also firms and tones each side of the body and helps to improve posture.

THE EXERCISE Sit on the floor, back to back, with your legs stretched open to the sides. Interlock your arms, as shown in the photographs.

Bring your bodies down first on one side, then on the other, elbows aiming to the floor between your bodies. Do this sequence 30 times to each side, stopping to rest for the count of 10 after each set of 10.

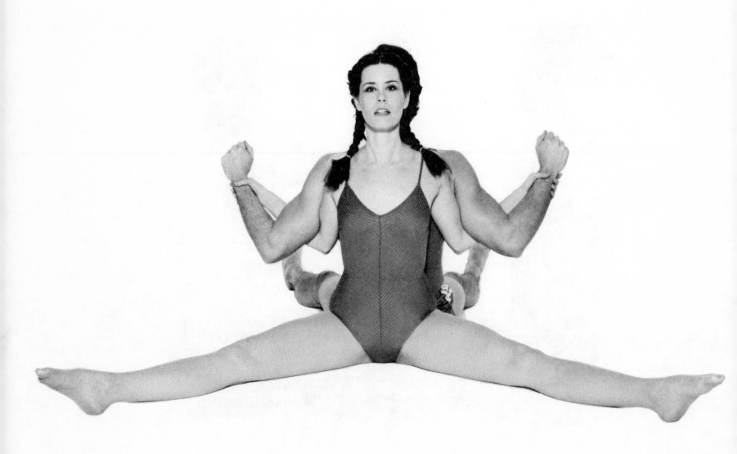

DOS AND DON'TS Keep your backs straight; don't tilt forward or backward. If you can't quite reach the floor, don't force it. Keep your abdomens tight and your rib cages lifted out of your hips. Pause and lift before you bend to the other side.

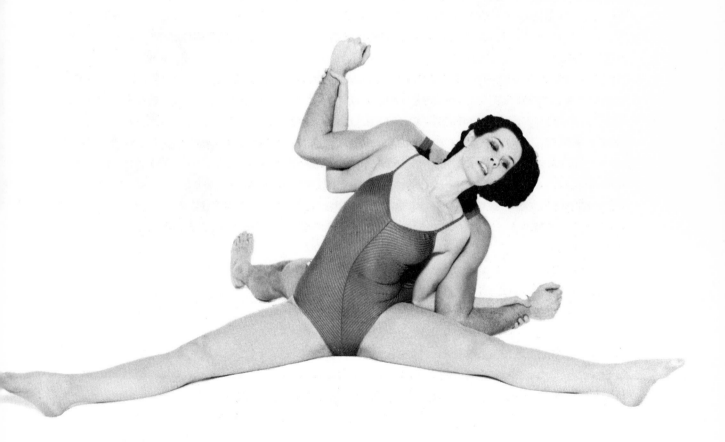

TORSO TWIST

BENEFITS This exercise firms, tones, and stretches the muscles in the chest, back, waist, and arms. It's also good for developing proper alignment and posture.

THE EXERCISE Sit on the floor facing each other with your knees bent and your feet tucked under each other's buttocks. Clasp your hands on the back of your heads, keeping your elbows out and high.

Lift up and away from your hips and twist your torsos, each of you bringing one elbow forward to meet each other's opposing elbow. Then twist in the opposite direction, bringing your other elbow forward to meet your partner's other elbow.

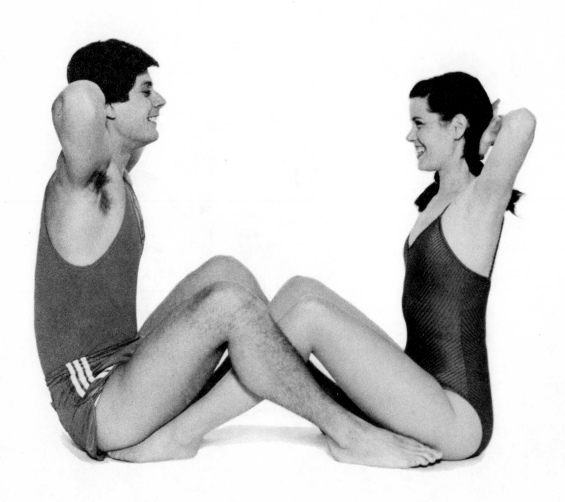

Do this sequence 30 times, stopping to rest for the count of 10 between each set of 10.

DOS AND DON'TS It's important to do this exercise with precision, so don't rush through it. Be sure to lift your rib cages up and out of your hips.

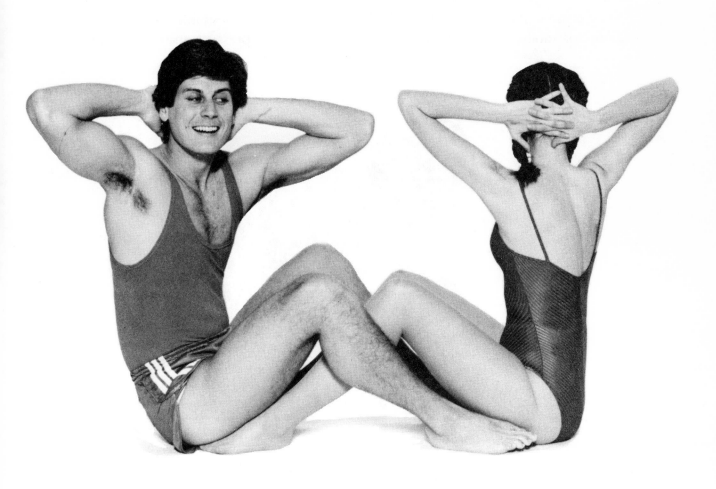

WRAPAROUND

BENEFITS This is an especially effective stretch for the legs, inner thighs, and lower back, with the added bonus of releasing tension in the neck, shoulders, and spine. It's a great way to get closer!

THE EXERCISE One of you sits on the floor, your legs stretched open to the sides. Your partner drapes his body over your back, bringing his knees to either side of your body, and gently and slowly presses your body to the floor using the full weight of his body. Give in to the pressure, breathing deeply and rhythmically. When you have achieved the full extent of the stretch, hold it for a count of 10. Your partner then releases the pressure and you both slowly come back to your starting point.

Reverse positions and repeat the exercise.

DOS AND DON'TS The partner applying pressure should take care not to force the stretch; this exercise should be done gently. The partner who is stretching should remember to breathe deeply. You can use your bodies to massage each other's spine. Each person's degree of flexibility is different; what is comfortable for one may be painful for another. Tell your partner when to apply more pressure and when to let up.

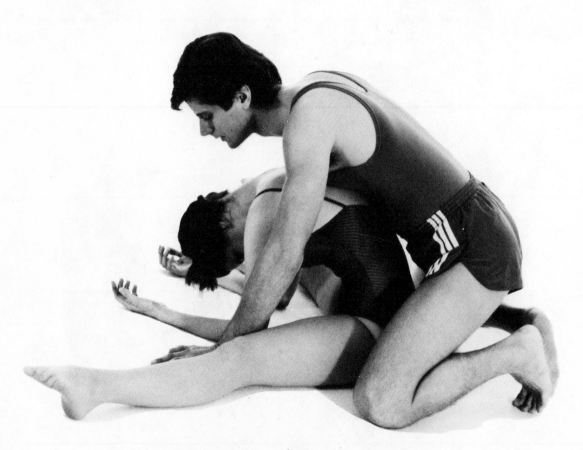

TWIST

BENEFITS This exercise is a terrific warm-up for the entire body. It also increases flexibility in the spine, hips, shoulders, and waist.

THE EXERCISE Sit facing each other, legs crossed, your knees overlapping, as shown.

Face away from each other and reach behind yourselves with your right hands to grasp each other's left wrist. With your left hands, grasp right wrists. Then gently pull away from each other to the left. You should feel a stretch in your right shoulders. Hold for a count of 10 and return to your original position with hands and wrists still engaged.

Repeat 3 times, and then reverse positions and do the exercise from the other side.

DOS AND DON'TS Keep your chests open and lifted, shoulders back. The twist is from the waist up; your buttocks and legs do not leave the ground.

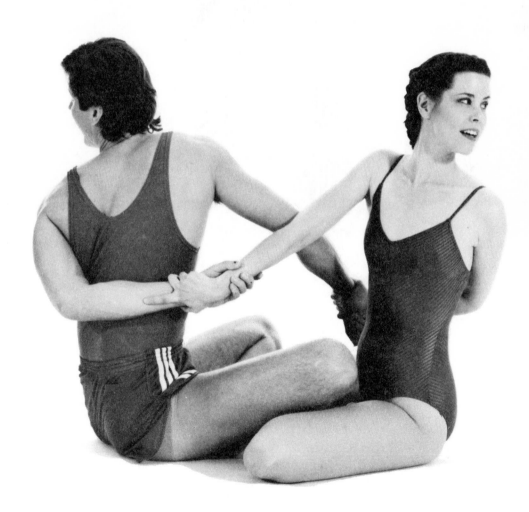

UP-DOWN SEESAW

BENEFITS This firms the stomach, strengthens the legs, and stretches the entire body.

THE EXERCISE Face each other in a standing position, holding each other's wrists. The shorter partner places her toes over the taller partner's toes and, standing tall, tightens her abdomen, legs, and buttocks. (If there is an extreme difference in your heights, stand about two feet apart instead.)

You will be alternating the movement, one of you remaining up while the other is down. One of you bend your knees and lower yourself as far as you can. Hold for

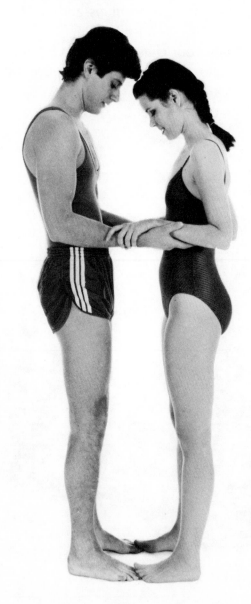

a count of 3, then slowly straighten up. Then you stand tall and tight as your partner lowers herself, holds for a 3-count, and straightens up.

Do this exercise 10 times, 10 up and 10 down for each of you.

DOS AND DON'TS Keep a firm grip on each other's wrists. Be sure to keep control over all parts of your bodies as you participate in each part of the exercise. Don't do the exercise so fast that you lose control!

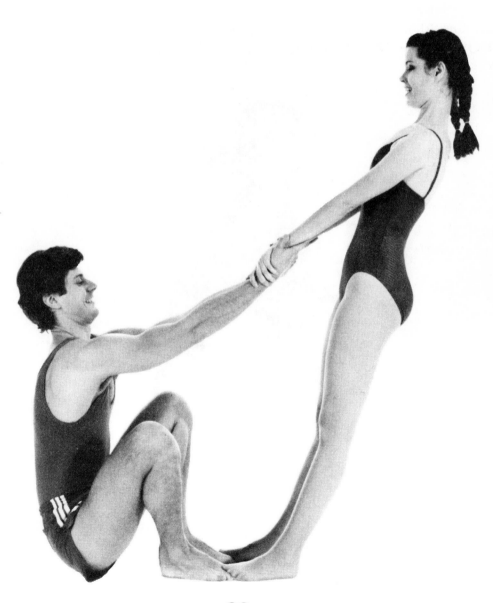

TOE TAP

BENEFITS This exercise will strengthen and stretch the feet and ankles, areas that are often neglected when it comes to exercise. The many people who suffer from weak ankles and aching, stiff, or swollen feet will get relief by doing this exercise.

THE EXERCISE Standing back to back about two feet apart, lean backward and press your upper backs against each other. Your feet should be firmly on the floor, legs slightly forward. Hook your arms through each other's, with your hands placed as shown in the photograph.

As you each press firmly against the other's back, first press your full feet to the floor and then, keeping your heels on the ground, lean back and flex the feet, lifting the toes as far as possible. Return toes to ground.

Do this 30 times, resting for a count of 10 after each set of 10.

DOS AND DON'TS Be careful not to bend your knees.

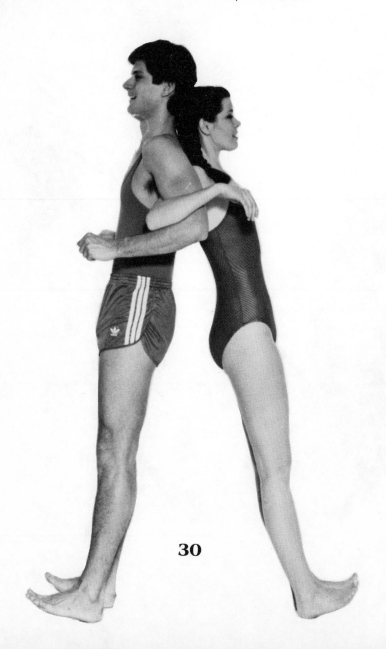

B. upper body exercises: arms, shoulders, chest, neck, and back

EASY Ⓔ	MEDIUM ⚠M	HARD H
Pendulum	Airplane	Butterfly
Backward Push-up	Windmill	Back Lift
Crisscross	Roundabout	Together Lift
Triangle	Up Lift	Tug
Inward-Outward Press	Push-out	Accordion
Lift	Bear Hug	Pump
Shrug	Locomotion	Pyramid Lift
Follow-up	Brick Wall	Together Again
Forward Hold	Inward-Outward	Cobra
	Press Too	Bottoms Up
	Together Cobra	Come Hither

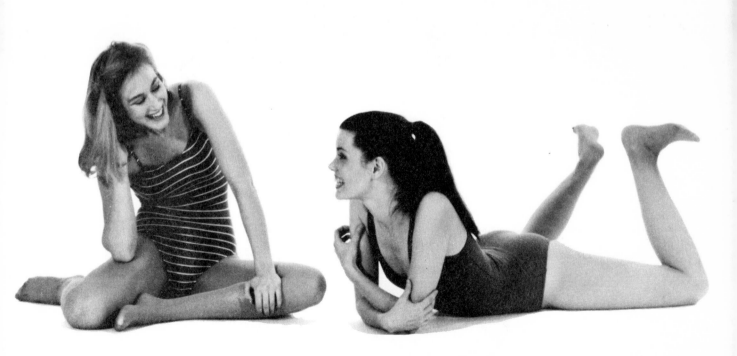

E PENDULUM

BENEFITS This exercise tones, firms, and strengthens the pectoral and arm muscles.

THE EXERCISE Stand facing your partner about a foot away. Both his and your feet should be a hip width apart.

Press the palms of your hands together, with your fingers pointing in opposite directions, as in the photograph. Be sure that your hands are at shoulder level with your elbows slightly lower.

Your partner reaches forward and presses in against your raised elbows. Try to separate your palms as he does this. Push out against his pressure for 3 counts, then relax for 3 counts. Do this exercise 3 times, then reverse roles and repeat.

DOS AND DON'TS Lock your arms, stand tall, and keep your abdomen tight. Exhale as you push out; inhale when you relax.

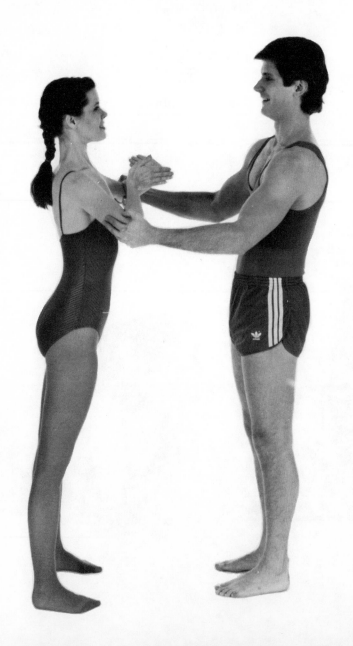

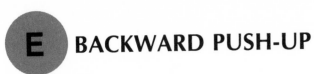 **E** BACKWARD PUSH-UP

BENEFITS This exercise aids flexibility in the chest and shoulders, as well as firming and toning the upper arms.

THE EXERCISE Stand with your backs to each other, far enough apart so that only your hands can touch when you reach back.

One of you place your palms on top of the other's. Push down as he pushes up for 3 counts. Release and rest for 3 counts. Do this 10 times. Then reverse hand positions so your partner pushes down as you push up.

Repeat this entire sequence 6 times.

DOS AND DON'TS Stand straight, don't bend forward, and keep your arms in close to your bodies. Keep your chests lifted up and out of your hips. Exhale on the press; inhale on the release.

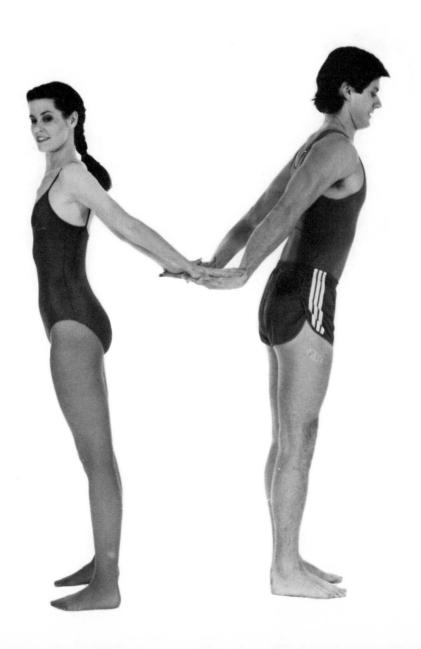

E CRISSCROSS

BENEFITS This exercise strengthens the arms and shoulders, and firms and tones the arms, shoulders, and chest.

THE EXERCISE One of you place your hands on top of the other's and press down while he pushes up. Without reducing the pressure, cross your hands over and then back again, as shown, moving them slightly upward each time you crisscross. After you have done this 10 times, your hands should be at face level. Then work your way back down again, crisscrossing hands as you do so.

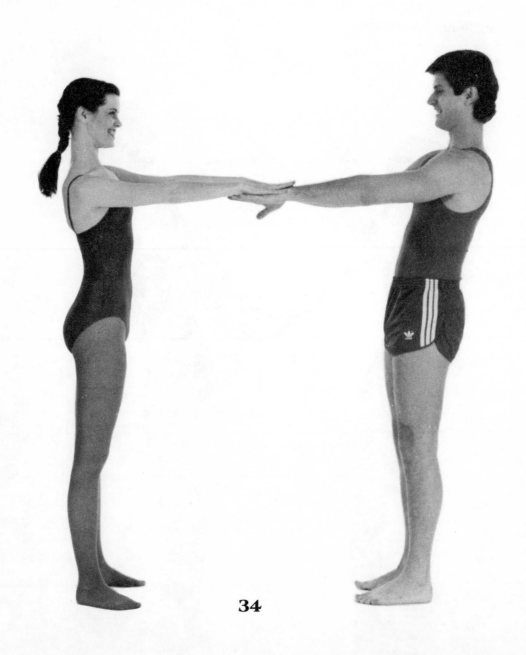

Switch hand positions, so your partner's hands are on top and repeat.

Continue until you have each had 20 times with your hands on top pressing down and 20 with your hands on the bottom pushing up.

DOS AND DON'TS Lock your elbows, stand tall, and really exert pressure on your partner's hands. Breathe normally; don't hold your breath at any point during the exercise.

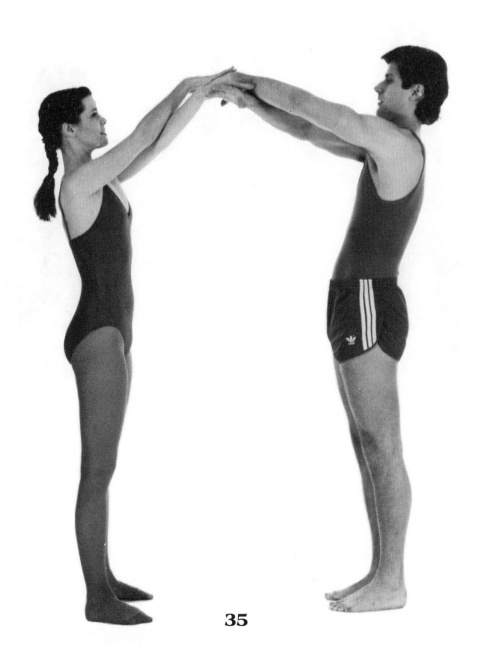

35

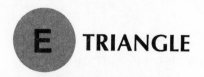

TRIANGLE

BENEFITS The thighs, calves and ankles will be stretched, strengthened, toned, and slimmed by this exercise.

THE EXERCISE Stand face to face, about four feet apart, a hip's width between your feet. Extending your arms out at shoulder level, press your palms firmly to each other's, as shown.

Lean forward until your forearms, from the elbows through the hands, are pressed against each other's. Keep your bodies rigid and your knees straight: There should be

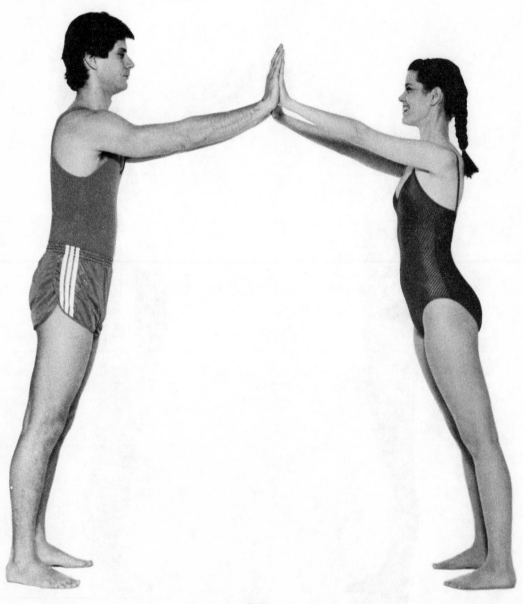

36

a straight line from your shoulders to your heels. Press as hard as you can and feel the stretch coming up through the back of your legs.

Hold this position for a count of 10, then push away. Repeat for a total of 10 times.

DOS AND DON'TS Keep your abdomens tight and your feet pressed on the floor. *Stretch*, don't strain. Breathe normally throughout the exercise.

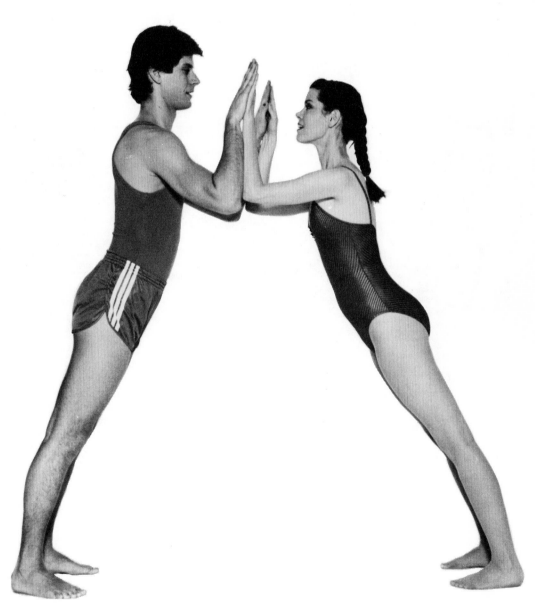

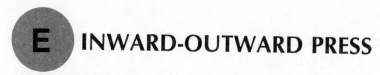

E INWARD-OUTWARD PRESS

BENEFITS This exercise firms and tones the arms and chest.

THE EXERCISE Stand facing each other, arms extended at chest level, with your palms pressed against each other's, as shown in the photograph.

Your hands should be on the outside, palms facing in; her hands should be on the inside, facing out. As she uses the full length of her arms to press her palms outward for the count of 3, you provide resistance with the full length of your arms. Then she releases for 3 counts.

Do 10 times, then reverse hand positions so you press out and she resists, and repeat another 10 times.

DOS AND DON'TS Both of you be sure to keep your chests and arm muscles tight. Lift your rib cages up and out of your hips. Do not lean forward. Breathe deeply; exhale as you press and inhale when you release.

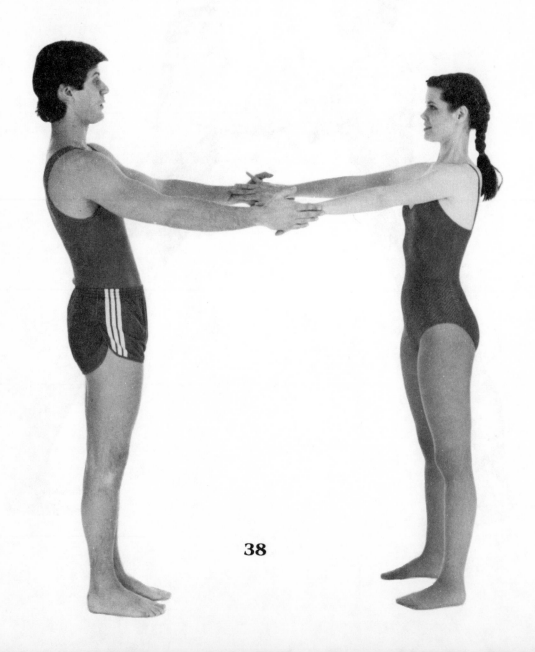

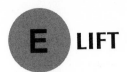 **LIFT**

BENEFITS Besides strengthening the entire arm, this exercise tones and gives a sleek graceful line to the upper arm and shoulder.

THE EXERCISE Stand facing each other one arm's length apart. One of you grasp the other's arms just above the wrist. His arms are hanging down at his sides, palms turned upward.

Provide resistance as he pushes his arms upward, bending them at the elbow, and bringing his forearms up to waist level. Continue to apply pressure as he lowers his arms.

Repeat this range of motion 30 times, resting for the count of 10 between each set of 10. Then reverse positions and repeat.

DOS AND DON'TS Don't rush through this exercise; it should be done in a slow and rhythmic motion. Stand tall, keep your chests high, and your rib cages lifted up out of your hips. Exhale as you push up; inhale as you lower your arms.

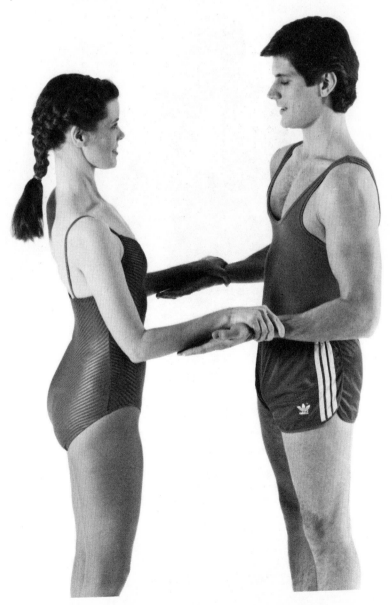

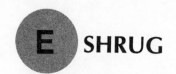 **SHRUG**

BENEFITS Besides releasing tension in your shoulders, this exercise firms and tones your chest, arms, and shoulders.

THE EXERCISE Stand back to back, holding hands, arms locked. Keep your feet a hip's width apart.

Together, pull down on both arms, then lift up one shoulder, release, then the other shoulder, release, then both shoulders together, and release. Rotate from side to side lifting one shoulder while lowering the other.

Do this 30 times with a 10-count rest in between sets of 10.

DOS AND DON'TS Move in a continuous motion with each other and don't allow your arm motion to be sloppy. Inhale as you lift; exhale as you release.

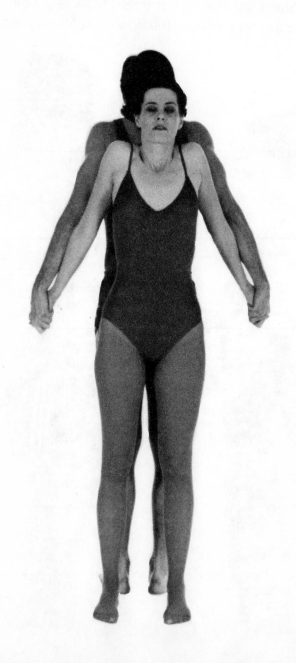

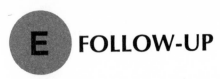 **FOLLOW-UP**

BENEFITS This exercise takes inches off the waist and hips. It also keeps the body flexible from shoulders through hips.

THE EXERCISE Stand with your backs pressed firmly together and your arms interlocked in a **T** as shown. Your feet should be about a hip's width apart.

Keeping your arms at shoulder height, twist your upper bodies around until at a ninety-degree angle to your lower bodies. Return to your original positions and then twist around to the other side.

Do this exercise 10 times to each side.

DOS AND DON'TS Don't force the twist. Be sure to keep your lower bodies stationary; move only from the waist up.

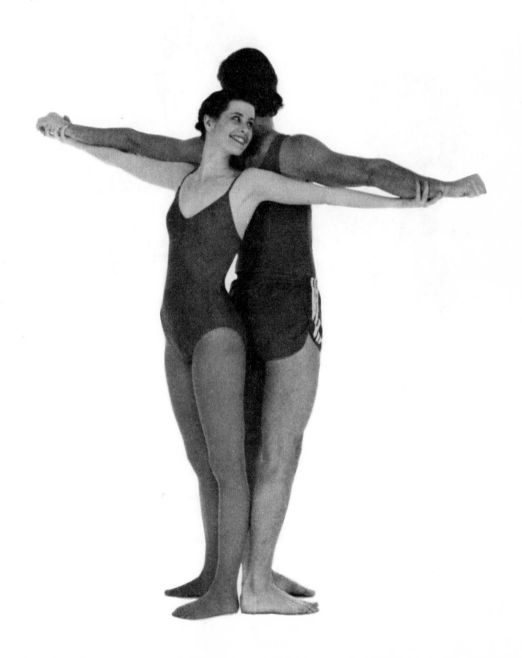

E FORWARD HOLD

BENEFITS This exercise strengthens the arms and shoulders and gives a firm, youthful look to the chest, arms, and shoulders.

THE EXERCISE Stand facing each other, arms outstretched in a T with palms against each other's.

Press palms for the count of 10, then release the pressure for the count of 5. Repeat this 3 times.

DOS AND DON'TS Keep your arms at shoulder level with both arms and palms centered. Be sure not to move your partner's arms toward him. Exhale on the push; inhale on release.

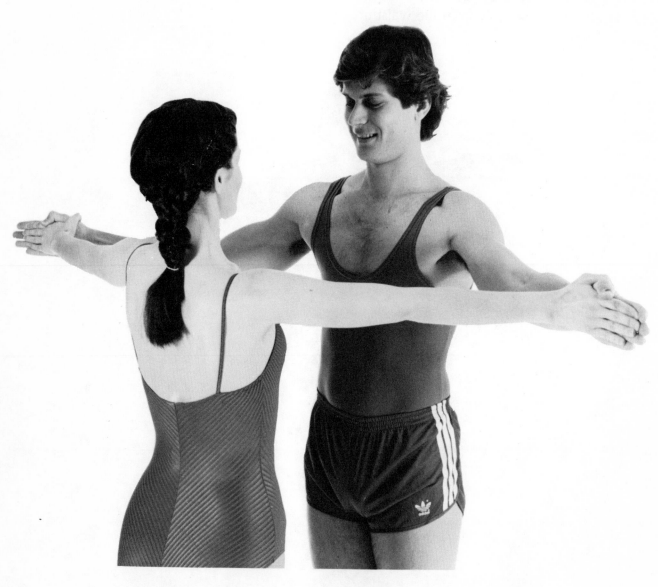

AIRPLANE

BENEFITS This exercise takes inches off the waist and hips and strengthens the chest, arms, and upper back. It also keeps the body flexible from the shoulders through the hips.

THE EXERCISE Stand with your backs pressed firmly together and your arms interlocked in a T. Your feet should be about a hip's width apart.

Keeping your arms straight, stretch down to one side as shown, then return to an upright position. Then stretch down to the opposite side; return. Next, one of you bend forward from the waist as the other arches backward; return. Then you arch backward as your partner bends forward; return.

Do a full circuit, all four directions, 15 times.

DOS AND DON'TS Don't rush; go through these movements smoothly and carefully. Breathe deeply and remember to keep your arms straight and your backs pressed firmly together.

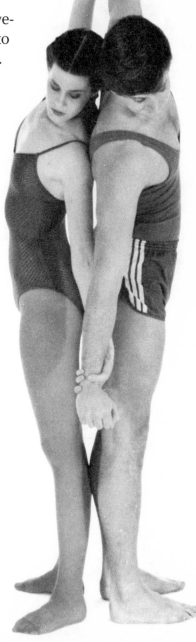

M WINDMILL

BENEFITS This exercise will warm and stretch the muscles in the upper arms and shoulders, making the area more flexible and firm. It also helps posture and lessens tension in the upper arms and shoulders. This exercise may bring relief to those who suffer from upper backaches.

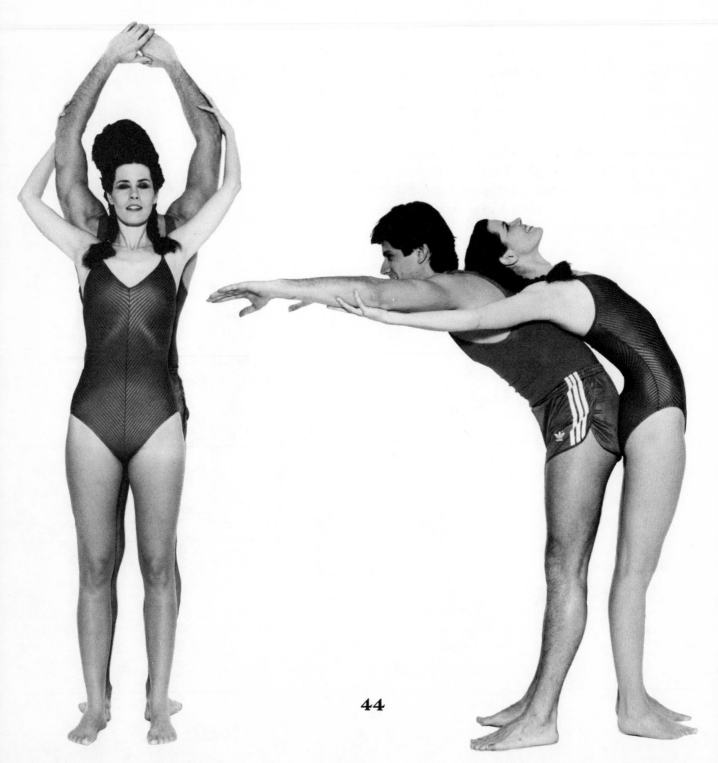

44

THE EXERCISE Stand back to back, your shoulders and buttocks touching. If you are approximately the same height, hold hands. If not, the shorter person can hold onto the taller one's wrists or forearms.

Raise your arms toward the ceiling, keeping them slightly curved, as shown. First one of you bend forward while the other bends backward with you. Pause, then you bend backward as your partner bends forward.

Straighten up, keeping your arms together and over your heads.

Then bend over to one side as far as you can. Come back up and bend over to the other side. Then come back up and bring your arms down.

Do this entire sequence 10 times at a rapid pace.

DOS AND DON'TS Make sure you lean neither forward nor back while raising your arms. When you bend forward and lean back, be sure your spine is relaxed and your back rounded. Keep your legs straight, your head up, and your chin out. Make sure that you are in total control of your movements throughout. If you're not, *slow down*! Breathe normally throughout the exercise.

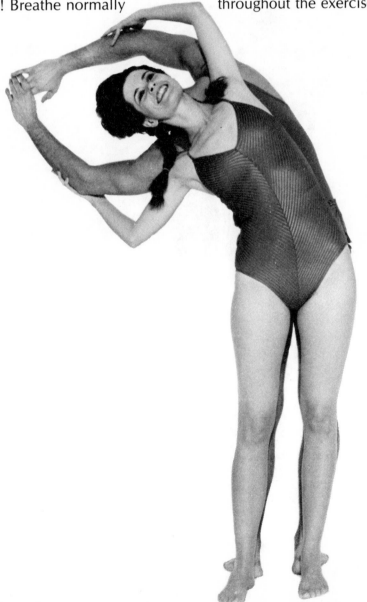

ROUNDABOUT

BENEFITS This exercise firms and tones the arms and shoulders. It also increases flexibility.

THE EXERCISE Stand back to back, arms outstretched in a T.

Grasp each other's hands and gently twist your torsos forward and then backward. Do 30 times in each direction with a 10-count rest between each set of 10.

Reverse hand positions and repeat. This time you resist as your partner twists his arm forward and back.

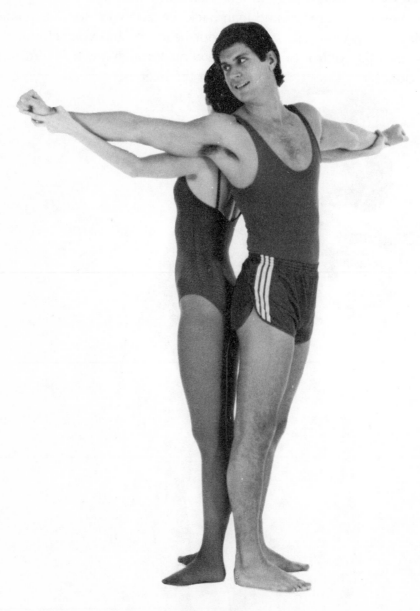

DOS AND DON'TS Don't allow your arms to drop beneath shoulder level. Stand tall and keep your chests high and your abdomens tight. Before you begin, decide which partner will establish the direction of the exercise. Breathe in rhythm with each twist.

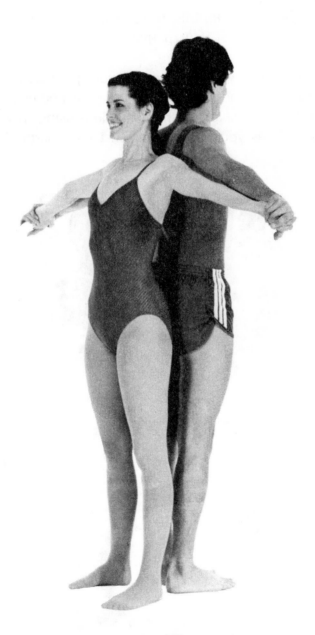

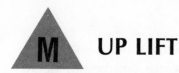

UP LIFT

BENEFITS While strengthening and firming the upper arms and chest, this exercise will also help to contour and uplift the chest.

THE EXERCISE Stand face to face, about one foot apart. Extend your arms to the sides at shoulder level.

One of you grasp the other's wrists and resist with all your arm muscles as he pushes against you. Release. Do this 30 times, resting for the count of 10 after each set of 10.

Reverse roles and repeat.

Variation: You might want to try this exercise with your arms rotated inward, so that when you are pushing against your partner, the back of your hand is pressing forward.

DOS AND DON'TS When you push against your partner, be sure to keep your chest and arm muscles taut. Stand tall. Don't press your bodies against each other's for additional strength. The entire exercise should be done using only the arm, shoulder, and chest muscles. Exhale as you push out against your partner's arms; inhale on release.

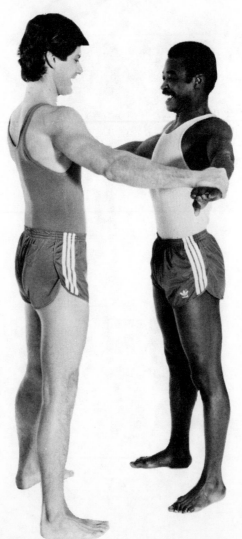

M PUSH-OUT

BENEFITS This exercise firms, tones, and strengthens the arms, shoulders, upper back, and chest.

THE EXERCISE Stand facing each other and bend forward to a flat-back position, letting your arms dangle freely.

One of you grasp the other's wrists and resist as she slowly pushes her arms out into a T. Then apply resistance as she slowly lowers her arms back to their original position.

Do this sequence 10 times, then reverse roles and repeat.

DOS AND DON'TS Each of you should keep your arms locked in a straight position. Tighten your stomachs, and don't hold your breath. Exhale as you push; inhale as you release.

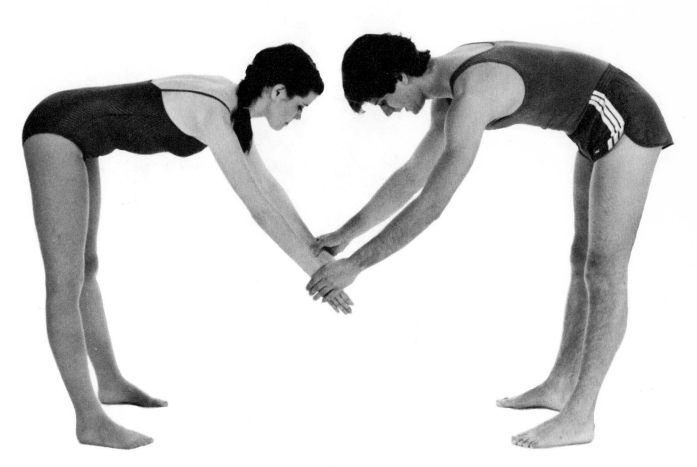

BEAR HUG

BENEFITS This exercise not only helps to achieve proper alignment and posture, it also firms, tones, and strengthens the chest, arms, shoulders, and abdomen.

THE EXERCISE Both of you face forward, one in front of the other. The one in front puts her hands on her shoulders, with elbows held high and pointing directly forward. Her partner's hands should be holding her forearms just below the elbow. Now she pushes her elbows out sideways against her partner's resistance, then releases.

Do this 30 times with a 10-count rest between each set of 10.

Reverse positions and repeat.

DOS AND DON'TS If one partner is much taller than the other, he or she can sit on a stool. The front partner should stand tall, with shoulders relaxed and a good lift through chest and rib cage. Exhale as you push; inhale as you release.

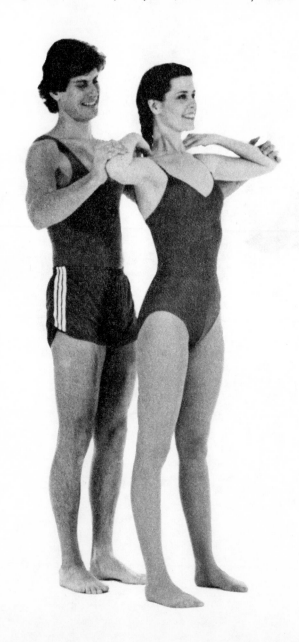

▲ LOCOMOTION

BENEFITS This is an excellent exercise for the neck and shoulders. Besides firming and toning, it releases tension and makes that area more flexible.

THE EXERCISE Stand facing each other, about two arms' lengths away, feet a hip's width apart.

Keeping your arms at chest level, bend your elbows and grasp each other's forearms. Lift one shoulder up toward your ear, roll it in a circle toward your back and then bring it forward. Repeat with the other shoulder. You should be moving your arms and shoulders in opposition to each other in a motion resembling the way old-fashioned train wheels moved.

Do 30 full circuits of your arms with a 10-count rest after each set of 10.

DOS AND DON'TS Your movements should be smooth and rhythmic. Keep muscle tension in your arms.

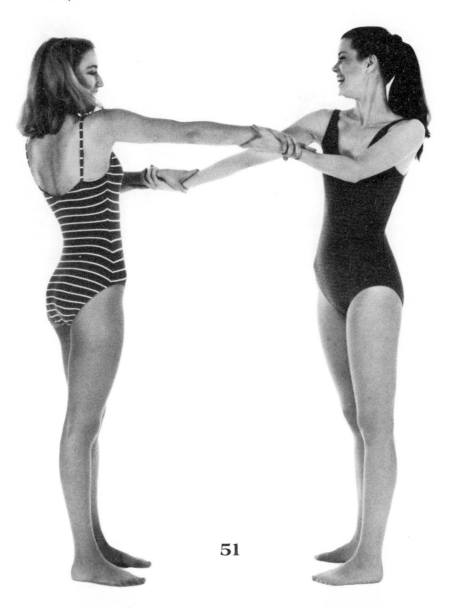

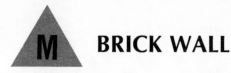

M BRICK WALL

BENEFITS Besides providing an excellent stretch for the legs and heels, this exercise strengthens the arms, chest, and shoulders.

THE EXERCISE Stand facing each other at a distance of about two feet. Both of you reach forward and press your palms against each other's, keeping your arms at chest level.

One of you bend one knee slightly and stretch the other leg out behind you while your partner remains standing straight. Then press as hard as you can against his hands while he resists. Hold the press for the count of 10. Reverse legs and repeat.

Then reverse roles and repeat the entire sequence.

DOS AND DON'TS Keep your abdomens tight and push with your chest and shoulder muscles. Breathe deeply; exhale as you push; inhale as you release.

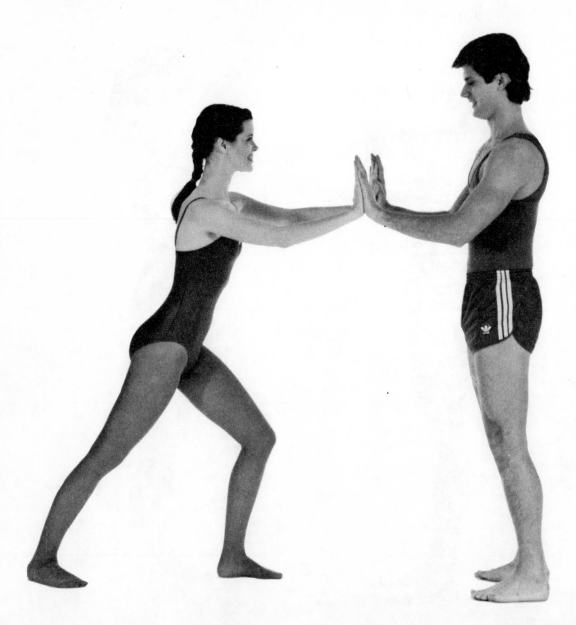

M INWARD-OUTWARD PRESS TOO

BENEFITS This exercise firms and tones the arms and chest.

THE EXERCISE Stand facing each other, arms extended at chest level, palms pressed against each other's, as shown in the photograph.

Your hands should be on the outside, palms facing in; his hands should be on the inside, facing out. As he uses the full length of his arms to press his palms outward for a count of 3, you provide resistance with the full length of your arms. Then he releases for 3 counts.

Do 30 times with a 10-count rest between each set of 10 press-releases.

Then reverse hand positions so she presses out and you resist.

DOS AND DON'TS Both of you be sure to keep your chests and arm muscles tight. Lift your rib cages up and out of your hips. Do not lean forward. Breathe deeply; exhale when you press and inhale when you release.

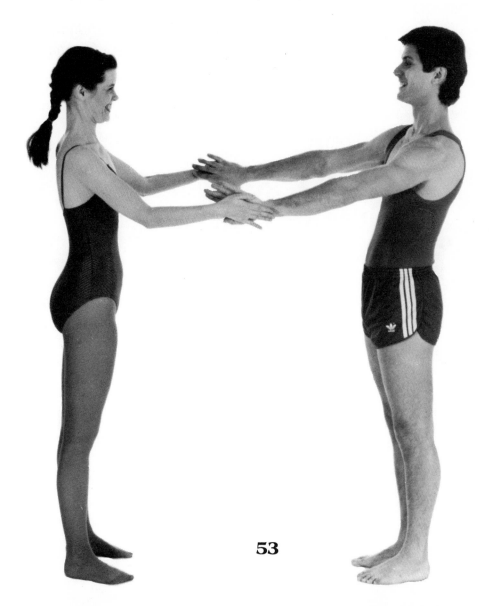

TOGETHER COBRA

BENEFITS This exercise releases tension in and strengthens the arms, shoulders, and chest. It also firms, tones, and strengthens the lower back.

THE EXERCISE Lie on your stomachs, facing away from each other, arms at your sides, foreheads on the floor. Your legs should be straight out behind you and intertwined as shown.

Slowly raise your heads, and then lift your shoulders and chests off the floor. Move your hands forward, placing them a few inches in front of your shoulders and, with their help, continue to lift, tilting your heads back as far as you can without discomfort. Continue lifting as high as you can through your torsos. Keep your shoulders and elbows relaxed. Hold your highest position for a count of 10, then gently return to your original position.

Do this exercise 3 times.

DOS AND DON'TS Try to do the movements in unison. Don't force anything, but do try to do the exercise in a controlled, relaxed fashion. Breathe normally throughout the exercise; do not hold your breath at any time. Keep your mouth and chin relaxed.

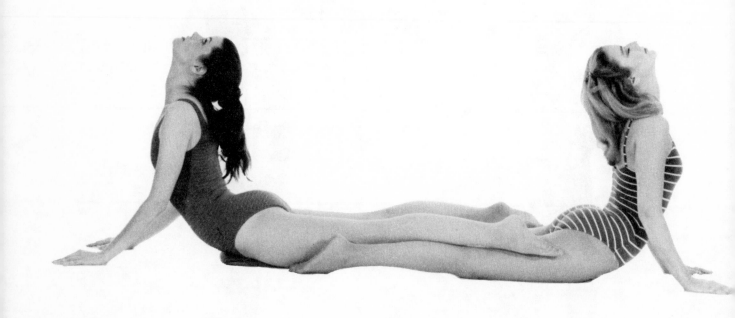

H BUTTERFLY

BENEFITS This exercise firms, tones, and strengthens the back, shoulders, and chest.

THE EXERCISE Lie on your stomachs facing away from each other, with your foreheads on the floor and your arms at your sides. Your legs should be intertwined as shown: your knees on the inside of his knees, your lower legs draped over his thighs.

Slowly raise your heads and shoulders to the count of 3 and then lift your arms, pointing them toward your feet. Now stretch your arms out to the sides in a T and take hold of each other's heels, as shown. Hold for the count of 3. Return your arms to their original position, then your head and shoulders to the count of 3.

Do this exercise 10 times.

DOS AND DON'TS Try to do the same movements at the same time as your partner. Exhale as you lift; inhale as you release.

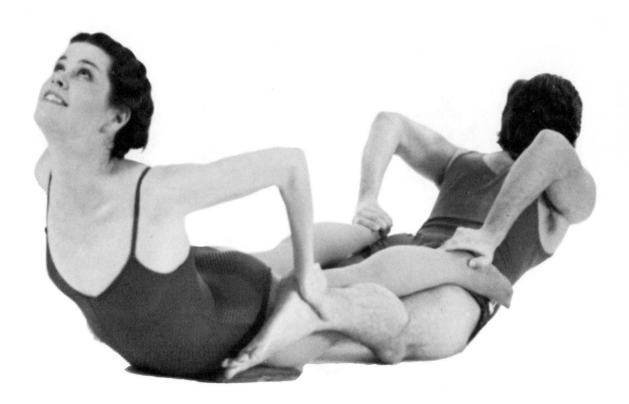

H | BACK LIFT

BENEFITS This exercise firms and tones the entire arm, and especially the fleshy part of the upper arm. It also serves as a terrific stretch for the entire body.

THE EXERCISE Stand facing each other two arms' length apart, then bend forward from the waist, bringing your heads down toward your knees and reaching up behind you with your arms.

Grasp each other's hands. Keeping your elbows locked, pull her arms toward your back; then let her pull your arms toward her back. As you do so, gradually bring your heads closer to your knees. Release and return to your starting position.

Repeat the sequence 5 times.

DOS AND DON'TS Don't pull too hard. Keep your abdomens tight and feel that stretch through the backs of your legs! Breathe deeply. If you exhale into the stretch, you'll find it easier to touch your knees.

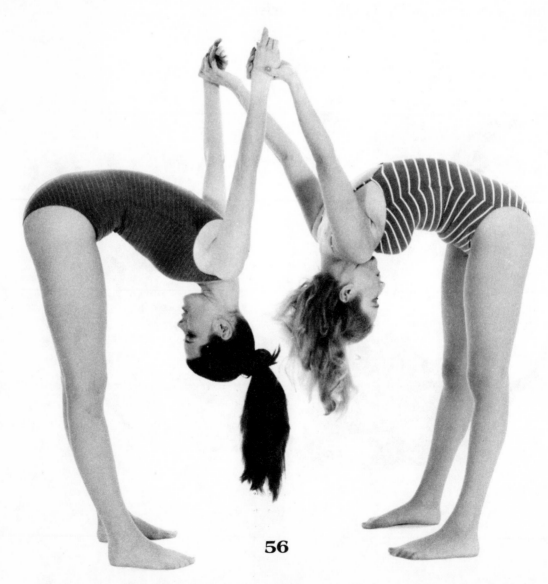

56

H TOGETHER LIFT

BENEFITS This exercise firms, tones, and strengthens the shoulders, chest, and arms.

THE EXERCISE Lie on your stomachs facing away from each other, arms resting at your sides, chins on the floor. Your legs should be intertwined as shown: your knees inside his, your lower legs on his thighs.

Raise your heads and upper bodies to the count of 5, then each of you swing one arm forward while the other arm grasps your partner's ankle, as shown. Lower, reverse arms and repeat.

Next, raise your heads and upper bodies and swing both arms forward. Hold for the count of 5. Lower your arms and relax.

DOS AND DON'TS Don't rush; remember to breathe deeply and exhale as you push.

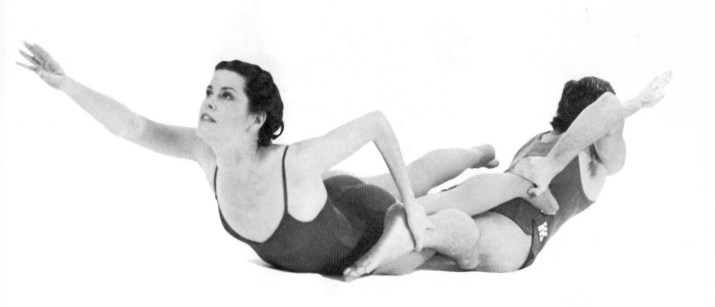

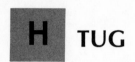

H TUG

BENEFITS Besides aiding flexibility through the body and shoulders, this exercise opens and stretches the rib cage, lifts and tones the chest.

THE EXERCISE Sit back to back with your legs crossed tailor-fashion.

Each of you raise your left arm and, bending it back behind your head, clasp your partner's right arm, which she has bent up from behind her back. Pull down on each other's left arms and hold for a count of 10. Then change arms and repeat.

Do this exercise 3 times on each side.

DOS AND DON'TS Lift your chests and keep your abdomens tight. Avoid rounding your shoulders or bending your heads forward. Breathe deeply throughout the exercise.

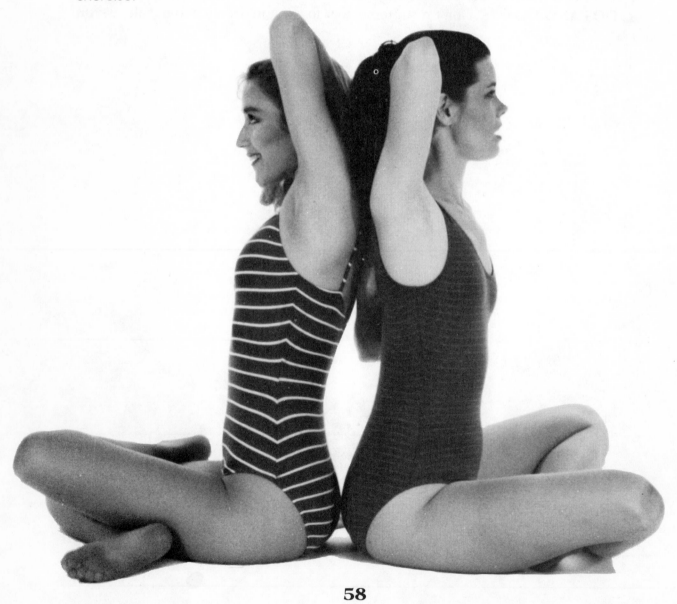

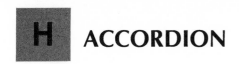

H ACCORDION

BENEFITS This is a wonderful strengthener for chest, arms, and shoulders.

THE EXERCISE Your partner lies flat on his back while you stand facing him, your feet tucked under his ankles. Keeping his upper arms on the floor, he reaches up with his hands and forearms and allows you to support your weight by pressing your hands down against his as you do 10 push-ups, keeping your back and legs in a straight line all the while.

Reverse positions and repeat.

DOS AND DON'TS Control and precision are most important in this exercise, so make sure you don't rush. The one who is doing the push-ups must remember to breathe properly: Exhale on the push-up and inhale on the release. Keep your back straight and abdomen tight while doing the push-ups.

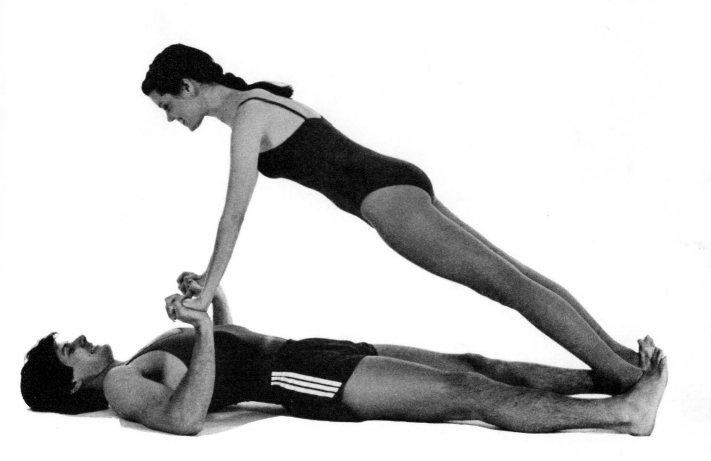

H PUMP

BENEFITS This is an excellent exercise for firming, toning, and strengthening the upper back, arms, chest, and legs.

THE EXERCISE One of you lie on the floor and pull your knees in toward your chest, the bottoms of your feet flexed so they point toward the ceiling. Your partner stands facing you with his feet about a shoulder's width apart. He then bends forward to a flat-back position and places his hands on your flexed feet, as shown.

As you push upward with your feet, your partner resists. When you have pushed all the way up and your partner's elbows have gone back and up as far as they can, he will push your feet back down as *you* resist.

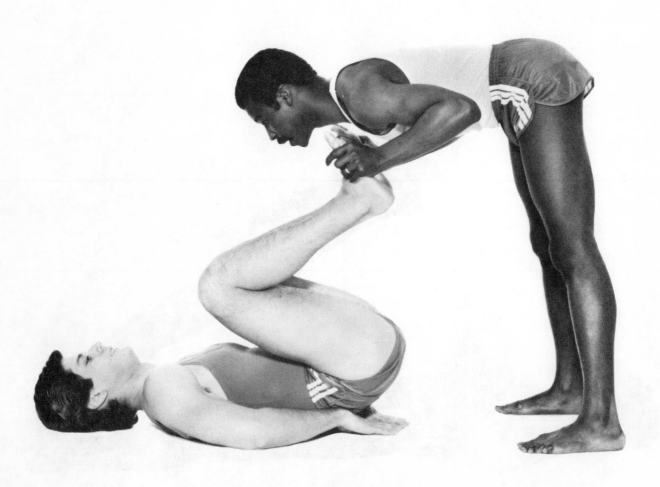

Do this exercise 30 times, resting for the count of 10 between each set of 10. Reverse positions and repeat.

DOS AND DON'TS The person who is standing up should move only his arms and be sure to use his chest and shoulder muscles to resist. Both of you must breathe properly (exhale to push and inhale to return) and keep your abdomens tight.

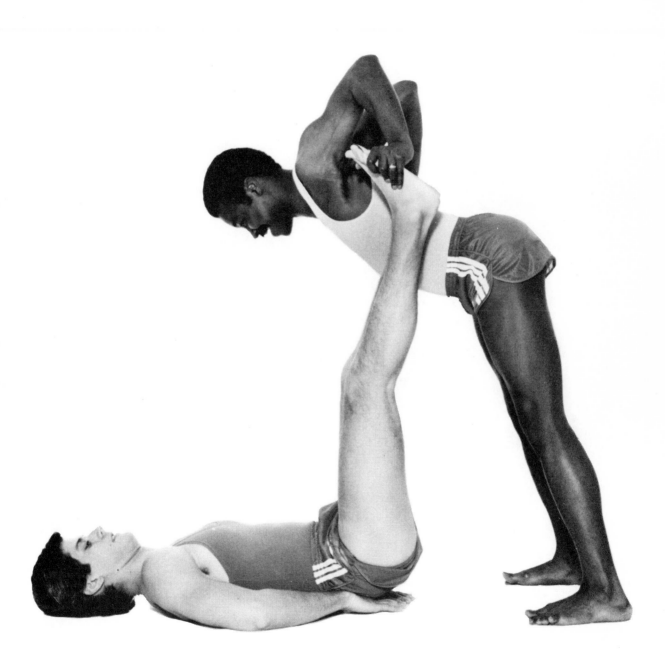

H PYRAMID LIFT

BENEFITS This exercise firms, tones, and strengthens the chest, shoulders, and upper back, as well as strengthening the lower back.

THE EXERCISE Lie on your stomachs facing away from each other, legs intertwined as shown: your knees inside his, your lower legs on his thighs.

Place your hands on the back of your heads and rest your foreheads on the floor.

Slowly lift your heads and shoulders, hold for a count of 10, and return to your original position.

Do this exercise 3 times.

DOS AND DON'TS Don't force the exercise, but try to lift and hold with control. Breathe properly: Exhale as you lift; breathe naturally as you hold; inhale as you come down.

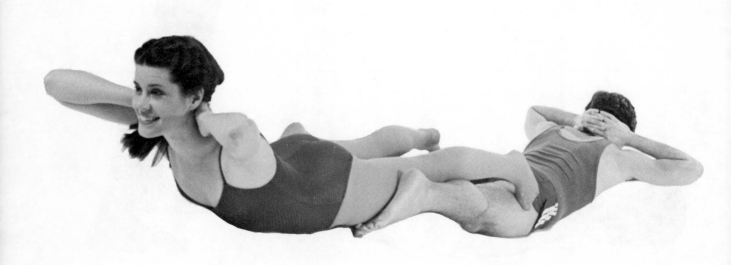

H TOGETHER AGAIN COBRA

BENEFITS This exercise releases tension in and strengthens the arms, shoulders, and chest. It also firms, tones, and strengthens the lower back.

THE EXERCISE Lie on your stomachs facing away from each other, arms at your sides, foreheads on the floor. Your legs should be straight out behind you and intertwined as shown.

Slowly raise your heads and then lift your shoulders and chests off the floor. Move your hands forward, placing them a few inches in front of your shoulders and, with their help, continue to lift, tilting your heads back as far as you can without discomfort. Continue lifting as high as you can through your torsos. Keep your shoulders and elbows relaxed. Hold your highest position for a count of 10, then gently return to your original position.

Do this exercise 6 times.

DOS AND DON'TS Try to do the movements in unison. Don't force anything, but do try to do the exercise in a controlled, relaxed fashion. Breathe normally throughout the exercise; do not hold your breath at any time. Keep your mouth and chin relaxed.

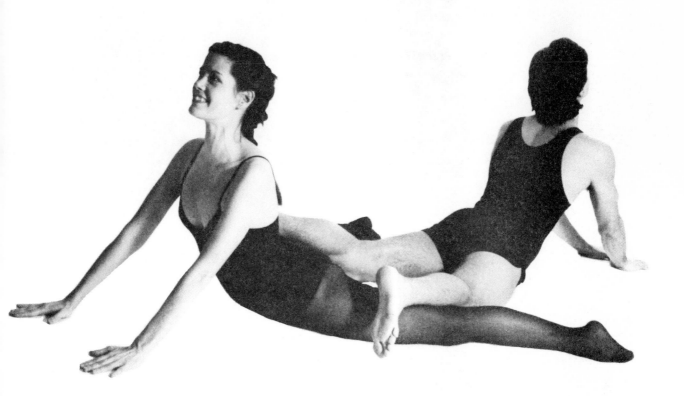

H BOTTOMS UP

BENEFITS This is an excellent stretch for the legs, feet, and heels. It also builds strength in the legs and helps with coordination and body alignment.

THE EXERCISE Stand facing each other, at arm's length. Your feet should be turned out as far as is comfortable, with your heels touching. Place your hands on each other's shoulders, as shown.

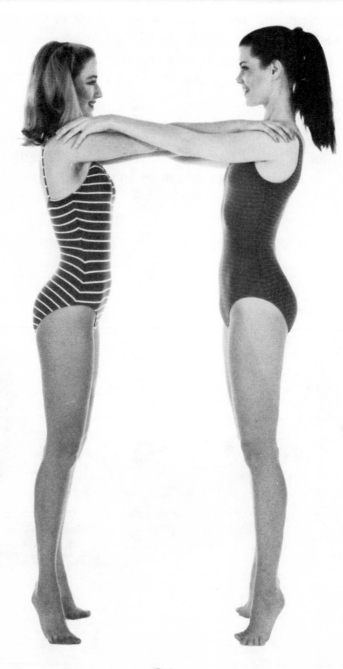

Rise up on tiptoe, then bend your knees and start lowering yourselves toward the floor. Stop when you have reached the squatting position shown. Hold that position for the count of 8, inhaling for the full count. Then press your heels down and stretch back up as you exhale.

Do this exercise 8 times.

DOS AND DON'TS Keep your bodies straight and lifted throughout the exercise. Be sure your abdomens are tight.

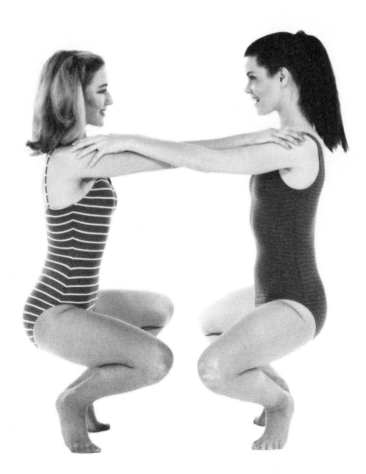

H COME HITHER

BENEFITS This exercise stretches the lower back and inner thighs while it tightens the abdomen and limbers the entire body.

THE EXERCISE Sit on the floor facing each other, your legs open to the sides. Reach forward and join hands.

One of you tighten your abdomen and pull back, lowering yourself as far back as you can while your partner gently rolls forward. Then roll forward as your partner pulls herself back in turn.

Do this exercise 30 times back and forward.

DOS AND DON'TS Remember to keep your abdomens tight. Be careful to pull your partner gently. Breathe normally and exhale into the stretch. If you are uncomfortable or the stretch becomes painful, let your partner know.

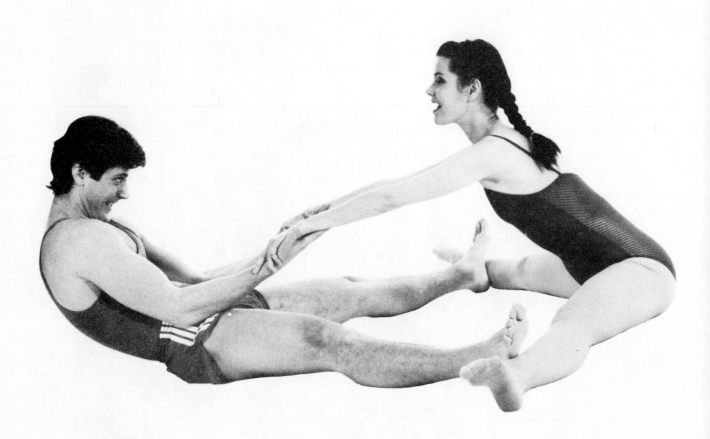

C. lower body exercises: midriff, waist, abdomen, buttocks, and hips

EASY (E)

Circle
Foot Push
Fold
Spring
Forward-Back
Easy Up
Leg-out
Big Push

MEDIUM (M)

Release Back
Climbing Foot Push
Fold Too
Bookends
Star Lift
Lean Back
Tilt
Piggyback
Leg-go-round
Bigger Push

HARD [H]

A Bicycle Built for Two
Curl-up Together
Blossom
Fold-over
Circle Too
Side Back Twist
Star Lift Too

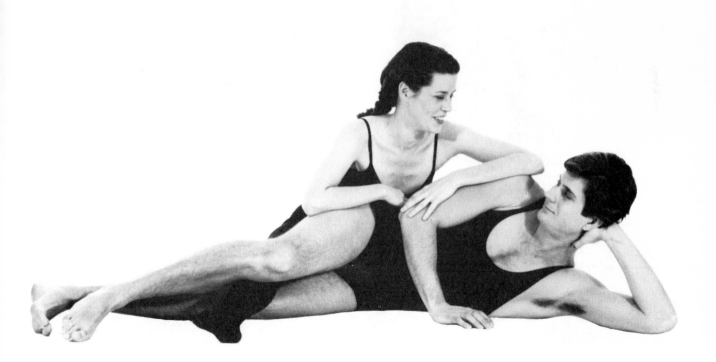

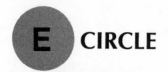 **CIRCLE**

BENEFITS This is an excellent exercise for trimming inches off the waist and hips. It also provides a superb stretch for these areas, as well as for the arms and shoulders.

THE EXERCISE Sit down beside each other, about two feet apart. Cross your legs tailor-fashion. Your inside hands rest on the floor next to each other's, as shown.

Stretch sideways toward each other, arching your outside arms overhead until you can grasp each other's wrist. Maintain your stretch while one of you gently pulls the other's arm sideways back toward the floor. Return to center but do not release your hold.

Do this 3 times, then reverse: She pulls gently and returns to center 3 times.

DOS AND DON'TS Don't allow your buttocks to lift from the floor; remain pressed through the floor as your bodies stretch sideways. Don't rush, but do maintain control. Do not lean forward or backward, only to the side. Breathe normally.

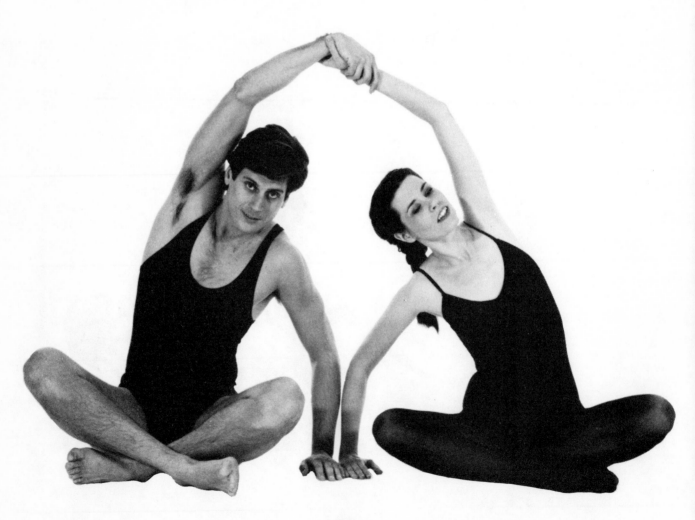

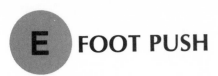

E FOOT PUSH

BENEFITS Besides improving balance and coordination, this exercise firms and tightens the abdomen and midriff muscles and strengthens and tones the legs.

THE EXERCISE Sit on the floor facing each other, bend your knees and draw them up into your chests. Reach forward and clasp each other's hands, balancing on your buttocks and pressing the soles of your feet against each other's soles.

Keep pressing your feet firmly against each other's feet while you both slowly straighten your legs upward. Hold tightly to each other's hands, tighten your abdomens, lift through your chests, and hold your position for the count of 6. Return to bent-knee, sole-to-sole position.

Do this exercise 3 times.

DOS AND DON'TS It's important to point your toes as you straighten your legs, keep your chins as high as possible, and breathe normally. Don't round your necks.

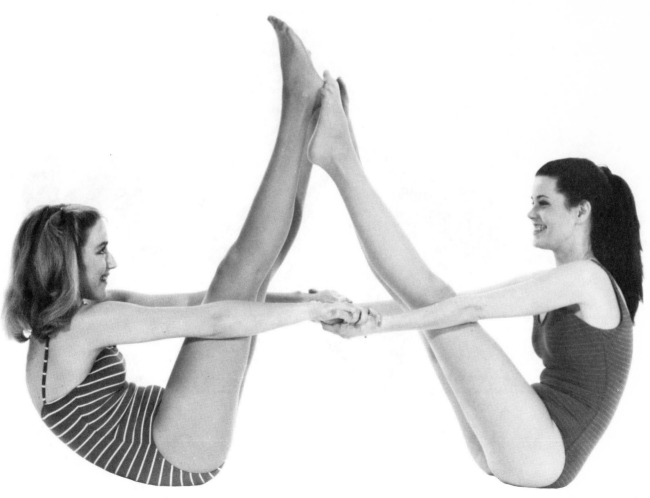

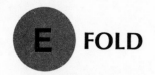

E FOLD

BENEFITS This exercise teaches balance and coordination as well as strengthening the abdomen. It also firms and tones the hips, legs, and abdomen.

THE EXERCISE Sit with your upper backs pressed firmly against each other's. Your feet should be on the floor, your knees separated and bent.

Reach forward and clasp your feet in your hands. Lift your feet off the floor and pull your knees into your chests. Hold for a count of 3, then lower.

Do this exercise 3 times.

Variation: If you are sufficiently limber, you can get a better stretch by reaching under your calves and holding your ankles, as she is doing in the picture.

DOS AND DON'TS Remember to keep your backs pressed firmly against each other's. Do the movements slowly and evenly. Breathe normally.

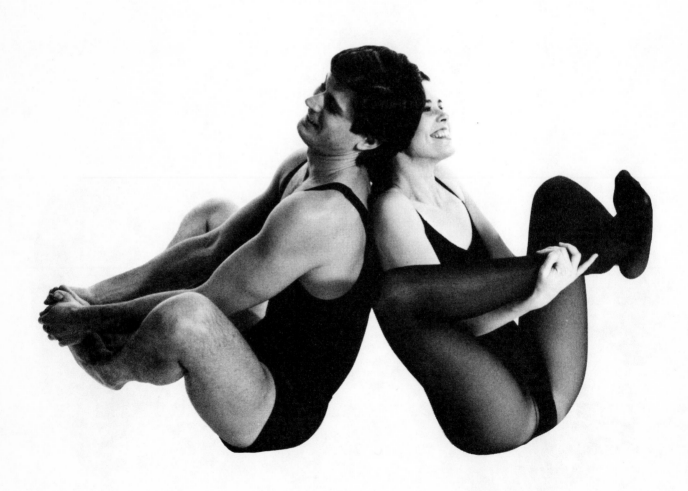

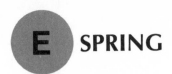

E SPRING

BENEFITS This exercise strengthens the midriff, chest, and upper back, while providing an intensive stretch for the entire body.

THE EXERCISE Stand facing each other with one foot on the other's toes, as shown, and clasping each other's wrists.

Together, lean back, allowing your arms to straighten and maintaining a straight line from head to heel. Hold for a count of 10, then pull back to an upright position.

Do this exercise 3 times.

DOS AND DON'TS Lean backward slowly and carefully to allow all of your muscles to stretch. Keep a firm grip on each other's wrists, straighten your elbows, tuck in your tailbones, and lift your chests. Breathe normally.

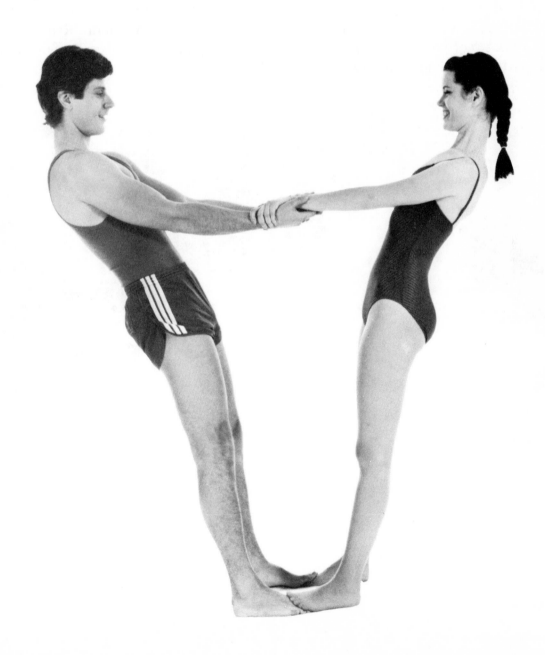

E FORWARD-BACK

BENEFITS This exercise firms and tones the abdomen while giving a terrific stretch to the legs. It is also a great tension releaser for the lower back.

THE EXERCISE Sit facing each other, your legs stretched out straight in front of you. Flex your feet and press your soles up against each other's. (If there is an extreme difference in your heights, the taller person can bend his or her knees.)

Reach forward and clasp hands. First one of you rolls backward, pulling the other with her and holds for a count of 10; then the other rolls backward and pulls her partner forward. Hold for a count of 10. Each of you should take care to keep your abdomen tight and your chin pressed in toward your chest throughout the exercise.

Do this exercise 10 times in each direction.

DOS AND DON'TS When stretching forward be sure to relax into the stretch. Don't force anything; do the entire exercise in a smooth, even motion. Remember to keep your feet pressed firmly against each other's. Inhale as you pull your partner forward; exhale into your forward stretch.

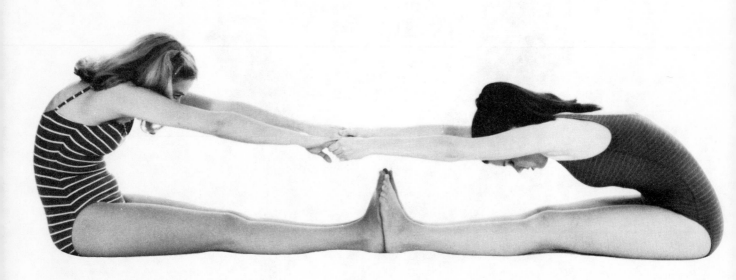

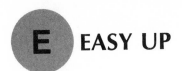

E EASY UP

BENEFITS This exercise strengthens the abdomen and lower back. It also firms and tones the midriff, abdomen, and arms.

THE EXERCISE Lie flat on your backs, facing away from each other, with your knees bent and feet pressed to the floor.

Place your legs as shown. Her feet should be pressed against his buttocks, his legs should be pressed against the outside of her legs. He presses while she pushes out with her legs.

Stretch your arms behind your heads and press your lower backs to the floor. Then, keeping your lower backs pressed to the floor, lift your arms, shoulders, and heads up from the floor and reach toward each other's hands. Hold that position for a count of 6 and roll back for a count of 6. Exhale as you lift up, inhale as you roll back.

Do this exercise 10 times. Then reverse leg positions and repeat 10 times.

DOS AND DON'TS Be sure to maintain pressure on each other's legs during the entire exercise.

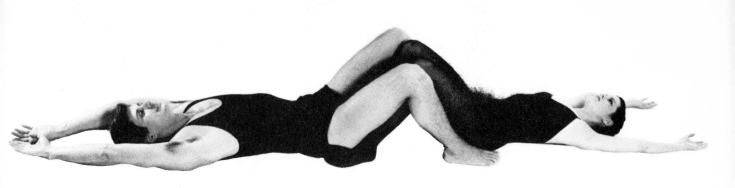

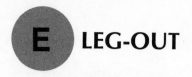

E LEG-OUT

BENEFITS Besides firming flabby thighs, tightening the abdomen and hips, and strengthening the legs, this exercise helps create balance and coordination.

THE EXERCISE Sit back to back with your upper backs pressed firmly against each other's. Your arms and hands are interlocked, the hands are on the floor, as shown.

Pull your knees into your chests, continue to press your upper backs firmly against each other's, tighten your abdomens, and then extend your legs out in front of you. Hold for a count of 10, then pull your knees back into your chests.

Do this exercise 3 times.

DOS AND DON'TS Do the exercise with control and be sure not to rush through it. Exhale with the lift; inhale as you release.

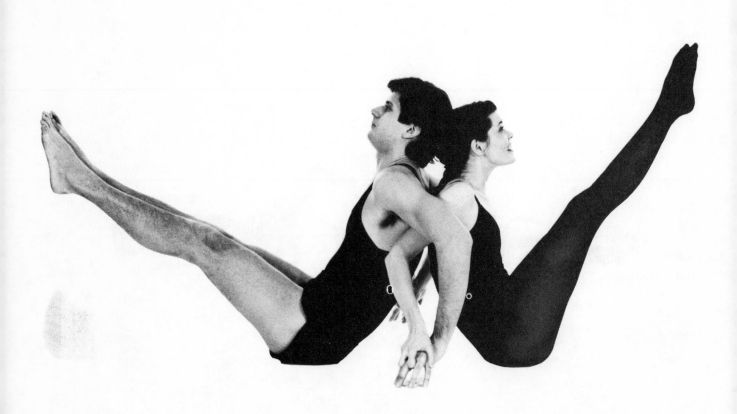

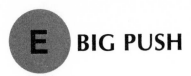 **BIG PUSH**

BENEFITS This exercise tightens and strengthens the leg muscles, firms and tones the abdomen and buttocks.

THE EXERCISE Lie on your backs facing away from each other with your buttocks pressed against each other's and your legs raised in the air at a right angle, as shown in the photograph.

Press your legs against each other's and push. Try to keep your legs at a ninety-degree angle to your bodies as you both do this. Push for a count of 10, then release and relax for a count of 10.

Do this exercise 3 times.

DOS AND DON'TS Remember to breathe naturally and to keep your legs raised at right angles to your bodies at all times.

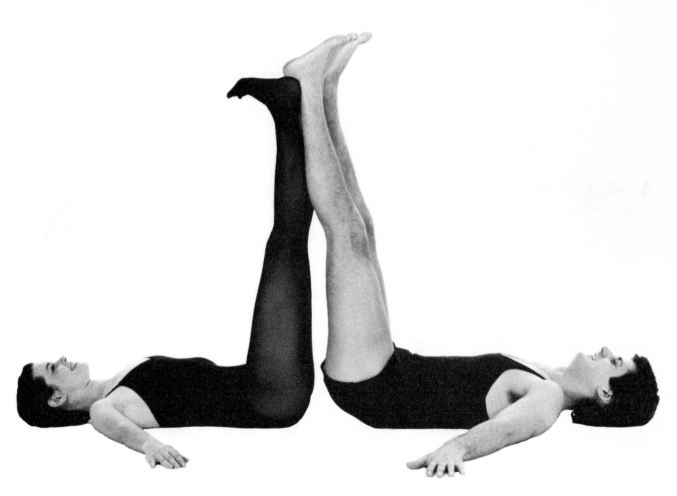

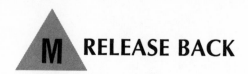

M RELEASE BACK

BENEFITS This exercise trims the waist and hips, and also strengthens the abdomen, midriff, and chest.

THE EXERCISE Sit facing each other with your knees bent. Each of you place your feet under the other's buttocks, press your chin into your chest, and extend your arms out toward your partner. Slowly roll back until your lower backs are on the floor. Press your lower backs into the floor, hold for a count of 6, and roll back up to your original position.

Do this exercise 10 times.

DOS AND DON'TS Stretch your arms out straight and keep them at shoulder level. Remember to press your lower backs firmly into the floor. Exhale as you roll back; inhale as you roll forward.

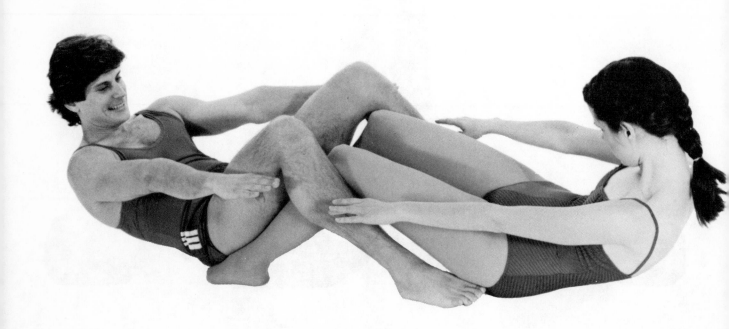

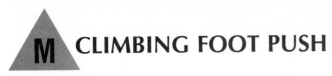

CLIMBING FOOT PUSH

BENEFITS Besides removing inches from hips and buttocks, this exercise strengthens the legs and helps with balance and coordination.

THE EXERCISE Sit facing each other, pull your knees into your chests, and press the soles of your feet against each other's soles at the same time as you reach forward and grasp each other's wrists.

Keeping your feet together, both of you push one leg and then the other up into the air, as shown.

Do this exercise 30 times on each leg with a 10-count rest between each set of 10. During your rest, push both legs up and rest in that position.

DOS AND DON'TS Do this exercise in a smooth, controlled, rhythmic motion. Keep your abdomens tight and breathe naturally.

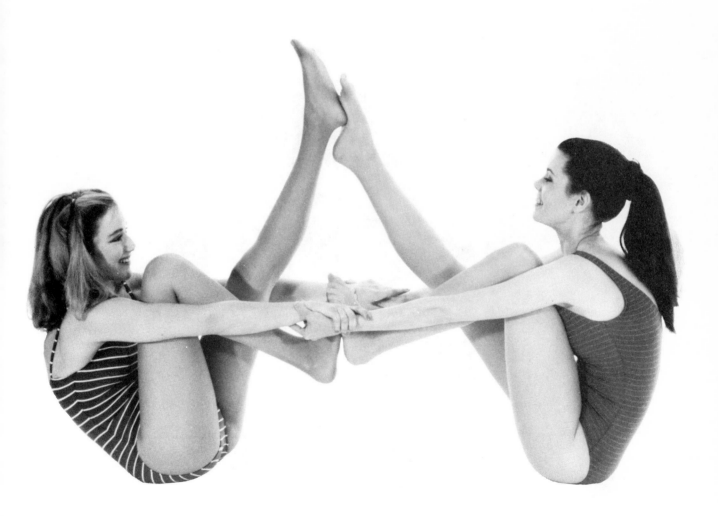

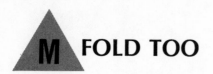

FOLD TOO

BENEFITS This exercise teaches balance and coordination as well as strengthening the abdomen. It also firms and tones the legs, hips, and abdomen.

THE EXERCISE Sit with your upper backs pressed firmly against each other's. Your feet should be on the floor, your knees separated and bent.

Reach forward and clasp your feet in your hands. Lift your feet off the floor and pull your knees into your chests. Hold for a count of 6, then lower.

Do this exercise 6 times.

Variation: If you are sufficiently limber, you can get a better stretch by reaching under your calves and holding your ankles, as she is doing in the picture.

DOS AND DON'TS Remember to keep your backs pressed firmly against each other's. Do the movements slowly and evenly. Breathe normally.

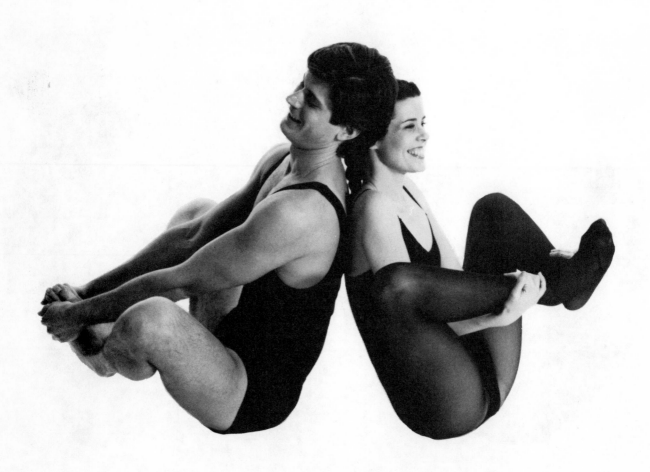

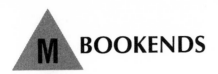 **BOOKENDS**

BENEFITS This exercise opens up the chest and shoulders and also tones from the neck and chest through the abdomen.

THE EXERCISE Stand facing each other, the less strong partner's feet over the other's, as shown. (If you are approximately equal in strength, each of you put one foot over and one foot under.)

Clasp each other by the wrists and lean back, straightening your elbows. Arch backward carefully, lifting your chests and keeping your heads back. Hold for a count of 10, then straighten and pull back toward each other.

Do this exercise 3 times.

DOS AND DON'TS Do this exercise slowly and smoothly. Be careful to keep a firm grip on your partner's wrists! Don't hold your breath. Keep your mouth and chin relaxed; don't strain your neck.

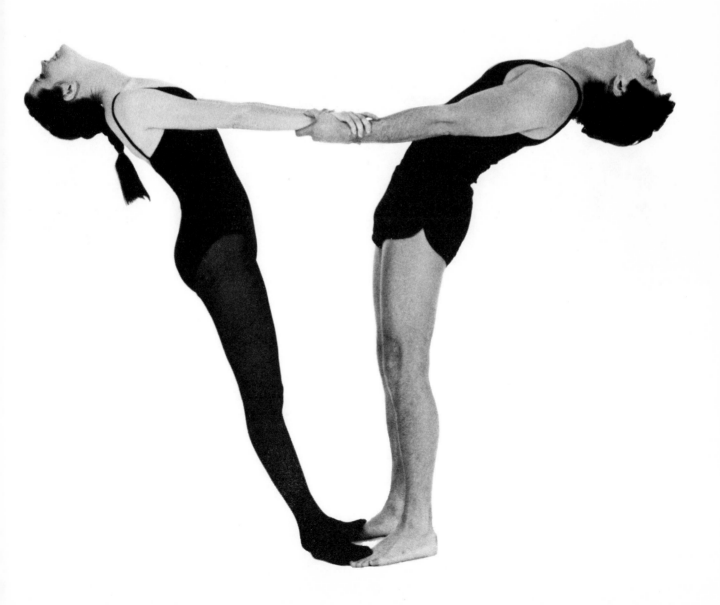

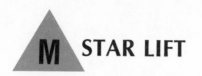 STAR LIFT

BENEFITS This is a very good exercise for strengthening the abdomen and lower back, as well as for firming and toning the midriff, abdomen, chest, and arms.

THE EXERCISE Lie flat on your backs, heads away from each other with your knees bent and your legs braced against each other, as shown.

Stretch your arms behind your heads and press your lower backs to the floor. Then lift up all the way, bringing your arms, heads, and shoulders upward until you are touching each other's fingertips. Hold for a count of 6, then pull your chins in toward your chests, and roll back down to the floor.

Do this exercise 10 times.

DOS AND DON'TS Control the exercise from a tight abdomen, but don't strain. Exhale as you lift and inhale as you roll back.

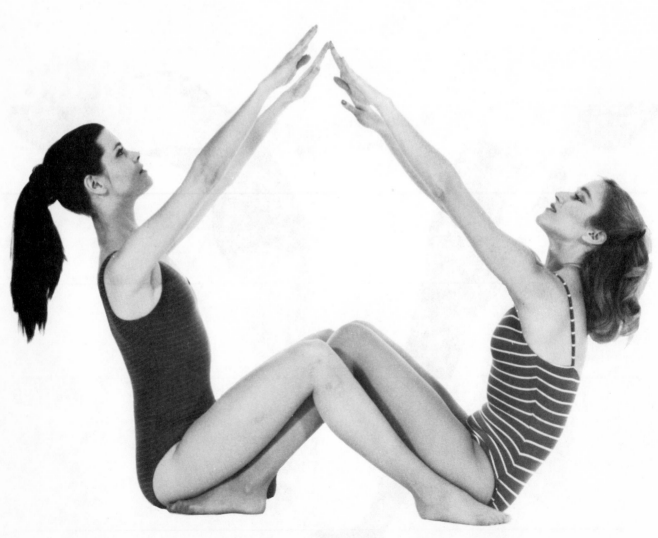

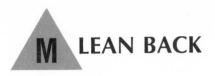 **LEAN BACK**

BENEFITS This exercise is a great strengthener for the abdomen, thighs, and buttocks. It will also improve alignment and balance.

THE EXERCISE Kneel facing each other, about one foot apart. Keeping your backs straight, raise your arms to shoulder level and clasp each other's arms above the wrist. Make sure your bodies are aligned: your rib cages lifted out of your hips, your chests high, and your abdomens, buttocks, and thighs tight. Lean slowly back as far as you can without losing this alignment.

Hold for a count of 5, then release your grips on each other's arms. Hold your arms outstretched for an additional count of 5, then clasp each other's wrists again and pull yourselves back upright.

Do this exercise 6 times.

DOS AND DON'TS Remember to keep your bodies straight and your rib cages up out of your hips. Breathe normally. Be careful not to lean back farther than you can control.

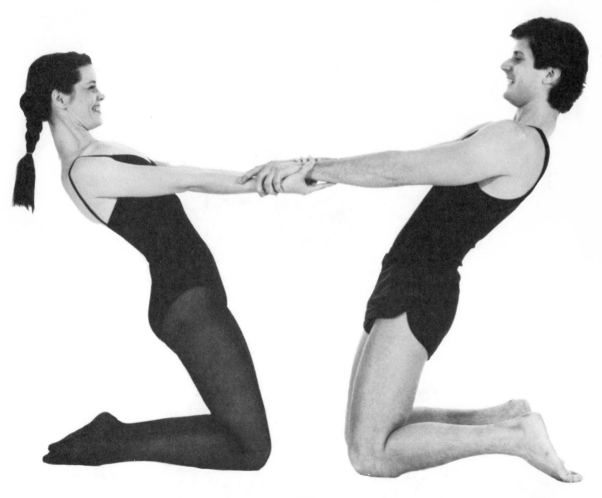

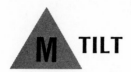 **TILT**

BENEFITS This exercise trims inches off the waist and hips as well as strengthening and toning the abdomen and legs.

THE EXERCISE Sit on the floor back to back with your arms out in a T. Your knees should be bent, your toes pointed and touching the floor, your heels up. Clasp each other's hands and pull your knees in toward your chests.

Twist your knees to one side while turning your heads and shoulders in the opposite direction, as shown. Move the arms in opposition so you face away from the ones that are raised and toward those that touch the floor. Return to starting position, then repeat on the same side.

Do this 30 times with a 10-count rest between each set of 10. Then repeat with your knees twisted over to the other side.

DOS AND DON'TS Keep your backs and shoulders firmly pressed against each other's. Don't rush through the exercise; maintain total control. Remember to breathe deeply and rhythmically.

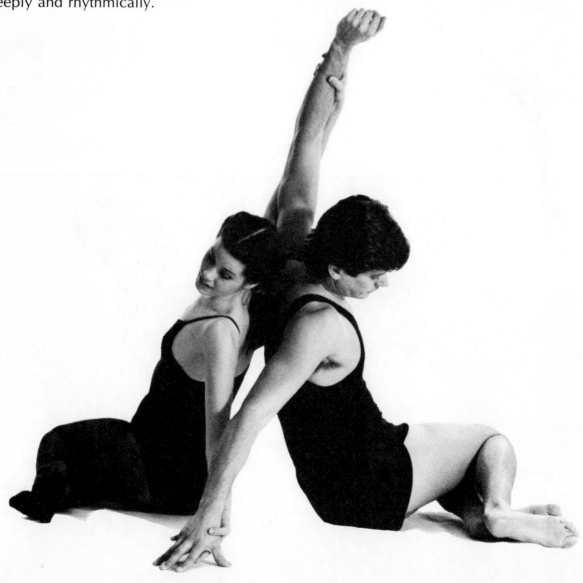

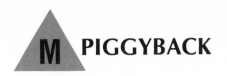

▲M PIGGYBACK

BENEFITS This exercise strengthens the abdomen as well as firming and toning the abdomen, hips, and inner thighs.

THE EXERCISE One of you sit on the floor directly behind the other with your knees bent, feet pressing on the floor, and your thighs placed against both sides of her body. The front partner should sit with her legs and arms stretched out straight in front of her.

Place your hands on the back of your head, with your elbows out to the sides. Contract your upper body and lower yourself only until your lower back is pressed on the floor. At the same time, your partner lowers her upper body backward as far as she can, contracting from her abdomen. Press your knees against your partner's body and pull your elbows in so they point frontward. Hold this for a count of 6, and then return to your original upright positions.

Do this exercise 6 times. Then reverse positions and roles and repeat.

DOS AND DON'TS Tighten your buttocks and hip muscles. Remember to breathe normally and keep your knees pressed firmly against your partner's body as you hold for the count.

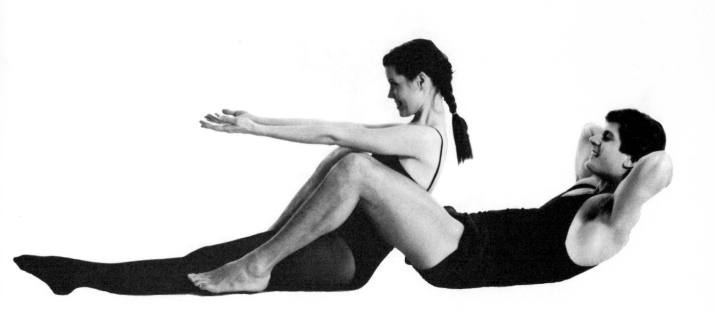

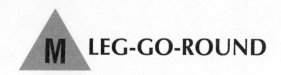

LEG-GO-ROUND

BENEFITS This is an excellent exercise for firming the legs and abdomen, as well as for building endurance.

THE EXERCISE Sit on the floor back to back, your upper backs pressed against each other's. Interlock your arms.

Stretch out your legs *straight* in front of you, holding them about three inches off the floor. Slowly bend your knees and pull them into your chests. Hold this position for a count of 3 while you inhale, then exhale, and then stretch your legs upward. Keeping your backs straight and your abdomens tight, hold this position for a count of 3 while you inhale, then exhale. Lower your legs until they are three inches from the floor. Inhale and repeat.

Do the entire sequence 6 times.

DOS AND DON'TS Keep your backs pressed against each other's. Each movement should be done in a smooth flowing motion and in unison with your partner.

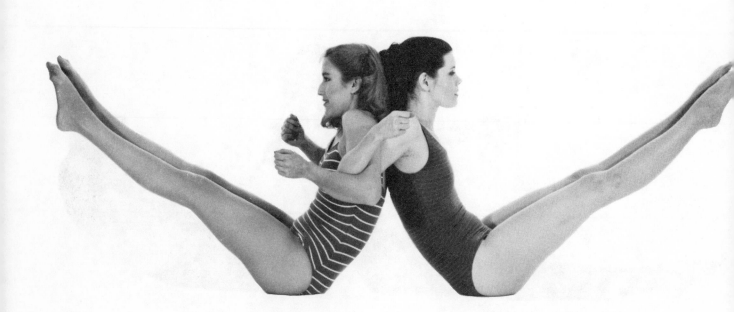

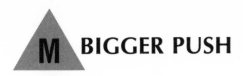

M BIGGER PUSH

BENEFITS This exercise tightens the muscles of the inner thighs, abdomen, and buttocks.

THE EXERCISE Lie on the floor, your buttocks against each other's, your legs straight up in the air and pressed against each other's. Press your arms out to the sides, keeping them on the floor.

One of you bend your knees slightly and press your feet up against your partner's legs, which should remain straight upright, feet flexed. Your partner resists your pressure. Keep pushing against his legs for a count of 10, then release.

Do this exercise 6 times, then reverse roles and repeat.

DOS AND DON'TS Keep your lower backs pressed to the floor and your abdomens tight. Maintain control over your movements and breathe naturally.

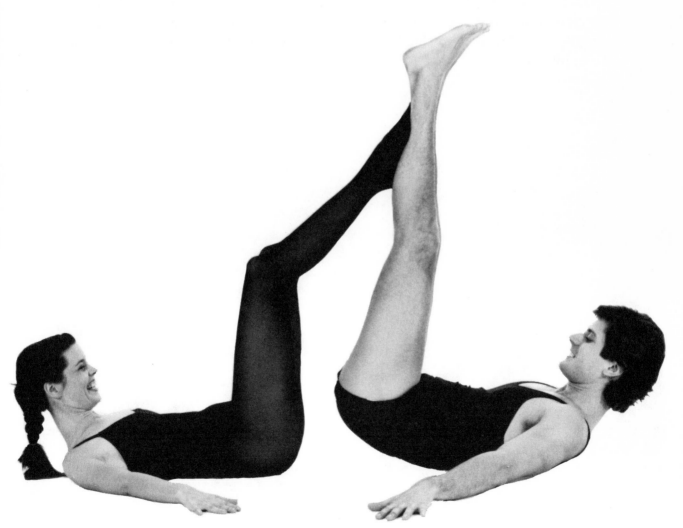

A BICYCLE BUILT FOR TWO

BENEFITS This is a fantastic abdomen strengthener and toner! It's also great for the legs, hips, and buttocks.

THE EXERCISE Lie on your backs facing each other, pull opposing knees in toward your chests, and push the other ones outward. The soles of your feet should be pressing against each other's, as shown. Place your hands on the back of your heads, with your elbows out to the sides.

Lift your heads and shoulders off the floor and try to bring your elbows forward and in toward each other, pressing your lower backs into the floor as you do so. Bend and straighten alternate legs in opposition to each other (like pedalling a bicycle) and twist your upper bodies toward whichever knees are bent.

Do this exercise 30 times forward and back with a 10-count rest between each set of 10.

DOS AND DON'TS Lower your heads and shoulders to the floor during each rest. Don't rush, keep your abdomens tight, and perform your movements with control and precision. The motion should be fluid yet rhythmic. Exhale as you push; inhale as you release.

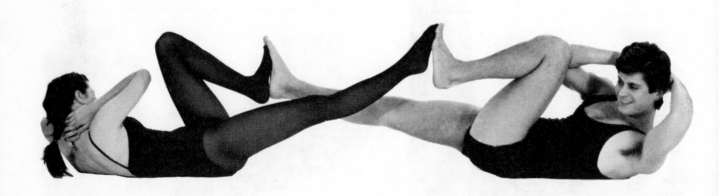

H CURL-UP TOGETHER

BENEFITS This is an excellent exercise for firming and strengthening the abdomen and is also beneficial for the chest and shoulders.

THE EXERCISE Lie flat on your backs, knees bent and braced against each other's bent knees, as shown, with your feet on the floor. Place your hands on the back of your heads, elbows out to the sides.

Keeping your lower backs pressed to the floor, lift your heads, shoulders, and upper backs off the floor, bringing your elbows forward and in. Then lower yourselves back down.

Do this exercise 30 times with a 10-count rest between each set of 10.

DOS AND DON'TS Keep your lower backs pressed against the floor, but don't strain. Be sure that your legs are locked and firmly pressed against each other's. Exhale as you rise and inhale as you go back down.

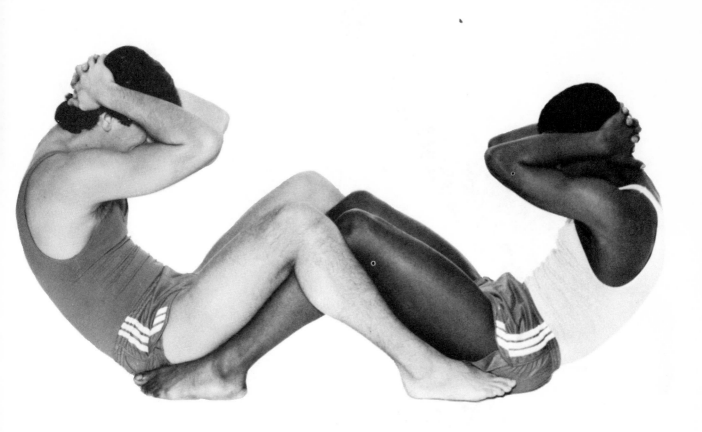

H BLOSSOM

BENEFITS This exercise is a terrific strengthener for the abdomen as well as a wonderful tension releaser. It firms and tones the legs, buttocks, hips, and shoulders too.

THE EXERCISE Lie flat on your backs, head to head, the tops touching. Stretch your arms out behind you and grasp each other's elbows, as shown.

Press your lower backs to the floor and lift up your legs, bringing them back over your heads until your toes are touching.

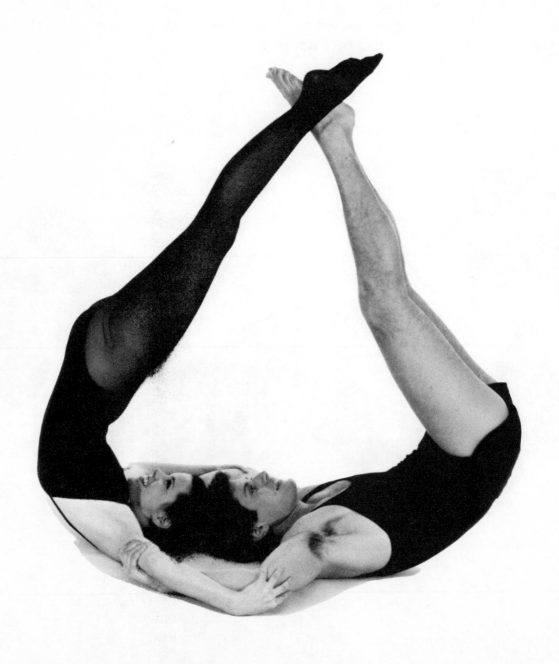

Balance for a count of 10, then continue bringing your legs over your heads until one of you is resting your feet on the floor, one on each side of your partner, and the other is resting his feet and legs on your buttocks, as shown. Relax and hold for a count of 10. Return to the legs-raised, toes-touching position and repeat.

Do this exercise 3 times. Do not start from the beginning; merely go back up to position 1, toes touching, from your relaxing position. After you have done the exercise 3 times, roll slowly back down to the floor along your spine, keeping your abdomens tight and your knees gently pressed down toward your faces.

DOS AND DON'TS Remember to keep your arms pressed to the floor. Control the exercise from your abdomens. Do it carefully and be sure not to rush through it. It doesn't matter which of you has his feet on the floor and which on the other's buttocks, but do decide in advance so there's no confusion.

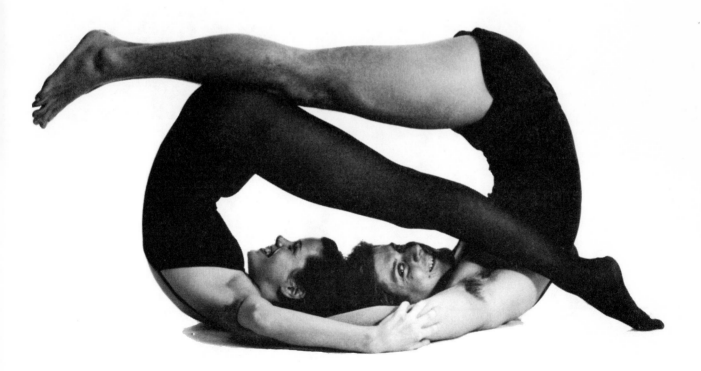

H | FOLD-OVER

BENEFITS Besides strengthening the legs, this exercise firms and tones the legs, hips, and abdomen.

THE EXERCISE Lie on your backs facing away from each other with your buttocks together and your legs raised in the air at right angles to your bodies. Press your legs against each other's and keep your feet flexed, as shown. Your arms should be flat on the ground, hands reaching toward each other's hands and holding them if possible. Your heads, shoulders, and backs should be pressed firmly to the floor.

One of you push your legs toward the other while she resists. When you have pushed as far as you can, hold your position for a count of 3, then reverse, your partner pushing your legs as you provide resistance. Again, hold the position for a count of 3.

Do this exercise 30 times back and forth with a 10-count rest between each set of 10.

DOS AND DON'TS To get the most out of this exercise, it's crucial to keep your abdomens tight and your backs pressed firmly to the floor. *Don't* strain.

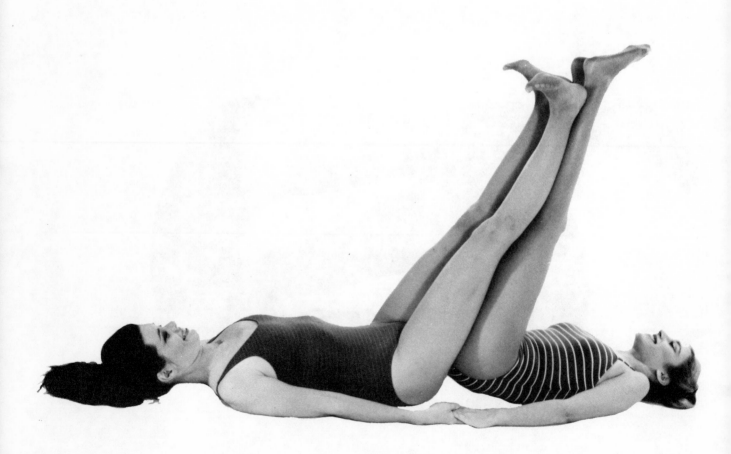

H CIRCLE TOO

BENEFITS This exercise trims and stretches your waist and hips and opens and firms your chest, arms, and shoulders.

THE EXERCISE Sit side by side on the floor about three feet apart. Stretch your inside legs toward each other, one of you pressing her foot against the other's leg. Both of you stretch your outer legs as far to the side as you can.

Propping your inside arms in back of you for support, as shown, lean your bodies toward each other. Arch your outside arms sideways over your heads toward each other and grasp hands or wrists. The partner whose foot is against the other's leg gently pulls back sideways toward the floor while her partner resists. Exhale to pull, inhale to release.

Do this exercise 10 times, then reverse foot positions and repeat, the roles reversed.

DOS AND DON'TS Be sure to lift through the chest and be careful to lean neither forward nor back.

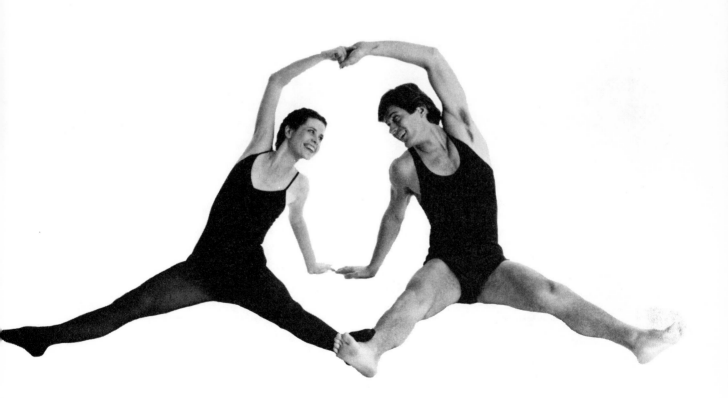

H SIDE BACK TWIST

BENEFITS Besides trimming and toning both sides of the body, as well as the abdomen and chest, this exercise strengthens the arms and shoulders.

THE EXERCISE Sit on the floor facing each other with your feet tucked under each other's buttocks. With your abdomens tight and your chins pressed in toward your chests, stretch your arms straight out at shoulder level.

Twist your bodies to the side in opposition to each other and roll back and down to your lower backs. Hold that position for a count of 6, then come back up, center yourselves again, twist to the other side, and roll down to your lower backs. Hold for a count of 6.

Do this exercise 30 times to both sides with a 10-count rest between each set of 10.

DOS AND DON'TS Be careful not to let your arms drop below shoulder level. Don't strain. Remember to keep your abdomens tight and your chins pressed inward. Exhale as you roll back; inhale as you roll up. Do not hold your breath at any time.

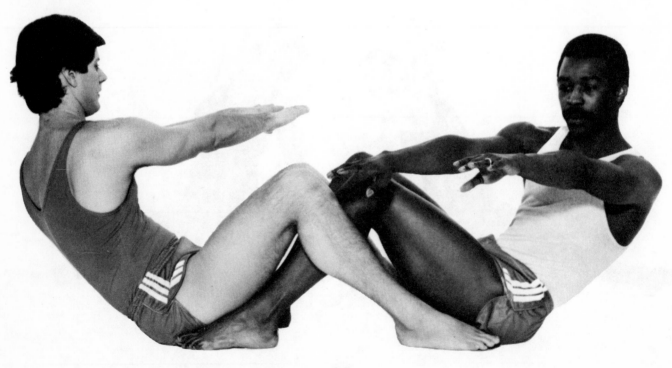

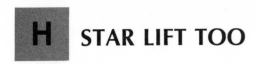

H STAR LIFT TOO

BENEFITS This is a very good exercise for strengthening the abdomen and lower back, as well as for firming and toning the midriff, abdomen, chest, and arms.

THE EXERCISE Lie flat on your backs, heads away from each other, knees bent, and legs braced against each other's, as shown.

Stretch your arms behind your heads and press your lower backs to the floor. Then lift up all the way, bringing your arms, heads, and shoulders upward until you touch each other's fingertips. Hold for a count of 3, then pull your chins in toward your chests and roll back down to the floor.

Do this exercise 30 times, with a 10-count rest between each set of 10.

DOS AND DON'TS Control the exercise from a tight abdomen, but don't strain. Exhale as you lift and inhale as you roll back.

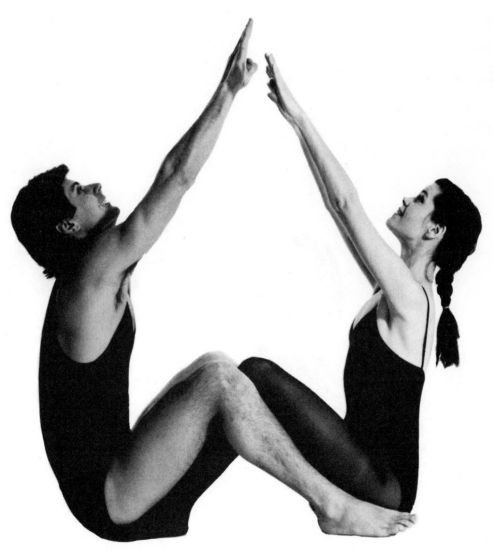

D. exercises for legs and feet

EASY (E)
Ankle Spread
Elevator
Knee Press
Rolling Knee Press
Bicycle
Under the Bridge
High Hip Press
Crossover
Stroll

MEDIUM /M\
Together Split
Leg Lift with Resistance
Hip Push
Bridge
High Kicker
Stroll Too
Thigh Lift
Swinging Palm

HARD [H]
Twisting T
Toe-Down Lift
Split Lift
Swan
Hip Lift with Friend
Sideways Pull
Thigh Lift Too
Hike

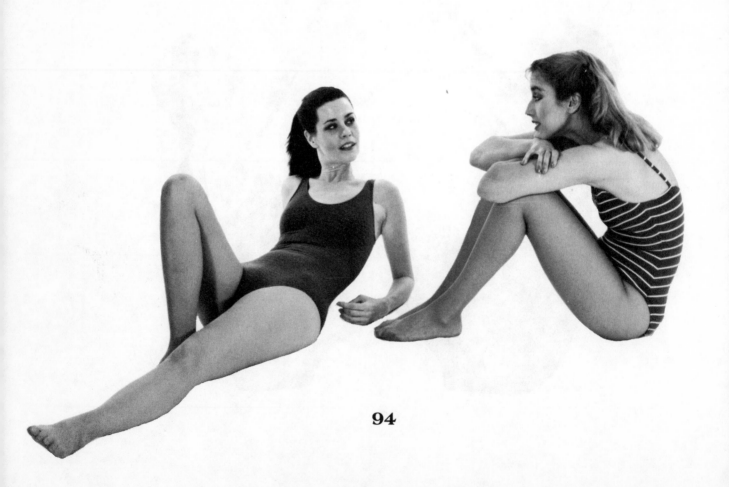

94

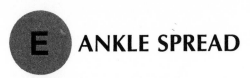

E ANKLE SPREAD

BENEFITS This exercise strengthens the feet, ankles, and calves, as well as toning and firming the entire leg.

THE EXERCISE Sit on the floor, legs outstretched toward each other, and lean back onto your elbows.

One of you put your flexed feet on the outside of the other's feet and ankles and provide resistance as she pushes against them by spreading her legs apart. She should be able to push your legs about a foot farther apart. At this point, maintain pressure and resistance while holding for a count of 3. Then release and return to starting position.

Do this exercise 10 times, then switch leg positions with your partner and repeat.

DOS AND DON'TS Neither of you should bend your knees at any point during the exercise. Don't push your partner's leg farther apart than twelve inches. Remember to continue pushing and resisting when you hold for the 3-count. Perform the exercise slowly and with control, breathing normally.

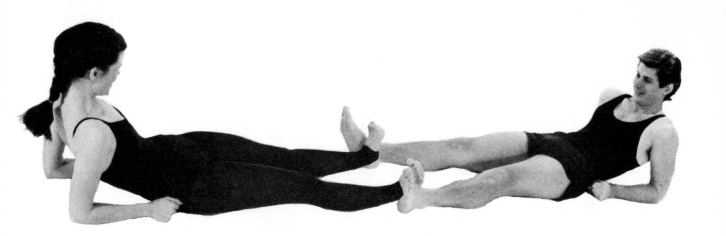

95

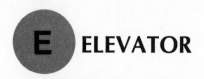 ELEVATOR

BENEFITS This exercise will stretch and firm the thighs, calves, hips, and feet, as well as slimming the waist and midriff. It builds strength and helps balance and coordination.

THE EXERCISE Stand back to back, feet together, and clasp each other's hands.

Rise up on your toes and, keeping your backs straight and pressed against each other's, bend your knees and lower yourselves toward the floor until you reach the position shown in the photograph. Hold for a count of 5. Come back up by pushing your feet against the floor and your backs against each other's. Hold this upright position (on your toes) for a count of 5.

Do this exercise 3 times.

DOS AND DON'TS Be sure to keep your knees over your toes and your torsos and spines straight. Keep your knees forward; don't turn them in or out. Exhale going down; inhale going up.

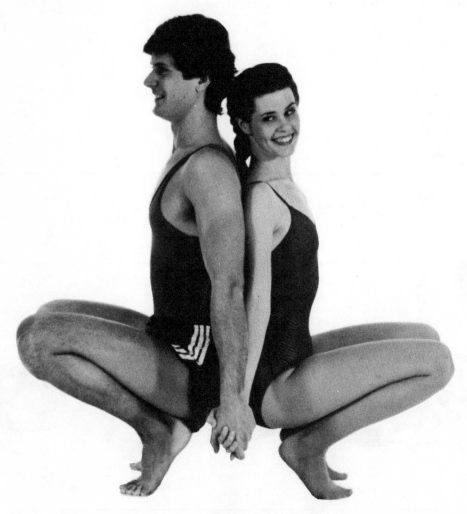

96

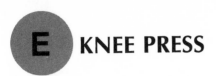

E KNEE PRESS

BENEFITS This exercise works the long muscles on the inside and outside of the thighs. It also tones, tightens, and strengthens the thighs.

THE EXERCISE Sit facing each other, holding your backs erect and your arms propped behind you as shown. Only your fingers touch the floor. Bend your knees.

One of you place your legs outside those of your partner, as shown. Try to squeeze your legs together as he resists by pushing out against your legs. It doesn't matter if your partner can't separate his legs since the benefits from this exercise come from pushing as hard as he can. Hold for a count of 6, then relax.

Do this exercise 3 times, then switch leg positions and repeat.

DOS AND DON'TS Remember to keep your backs erect.

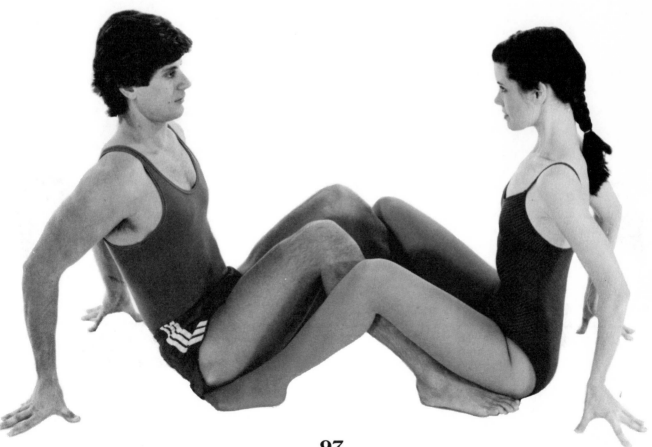

97

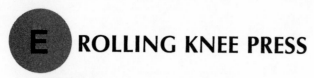

E ROLLING KNEE PRESS

BENEFITS This exercise firms and tones the legs and thighs, and also firms and strengthens the abdomen.

THE EXERCISE Sit facing each other with your knees bent. One of you place your legs outside the other's.

Squeeze inward on her legs as she presses out. Keep doing this as you both round your upper bodies and roll backward until your upper backs are pressed to the floor, as shown. Extend your arms toward each other, keeping them parallel to the floor. Hold for a count of 10. Then reverse leg positions and repeat.

Do this exercise 3 times.

DOS AND DON'TS Maintain constant pressure on the legs throughout. Remember to breathe properly: Exhale as you press your lower backs into the floor; inhale as you roll up.

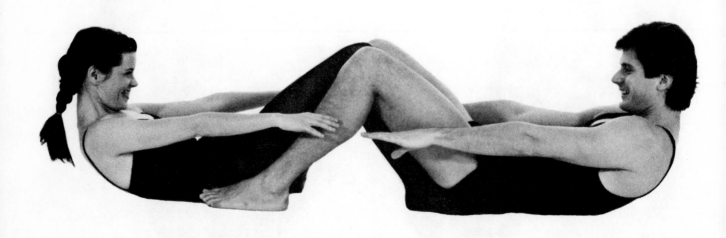

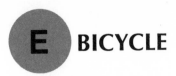

E BICYCLE

BENEFITS This exercise strengthens the legs, trims inches off the thighs and hips, and creates flexibility in all these areas.

THE EXERCISE Lie on your backs facing each other and supporting your upper bodies on your elbows, as shown. Lift up your legs and place the soles of your feet against each other's soles. Push against each other's feet, alternating in opposition in a pedalling motion. When one leg is fully extended, the other is back up against your chest.

Do this exercise 10 times.

DOS AND DON'TS Synchronize your breathing with your leg movements.

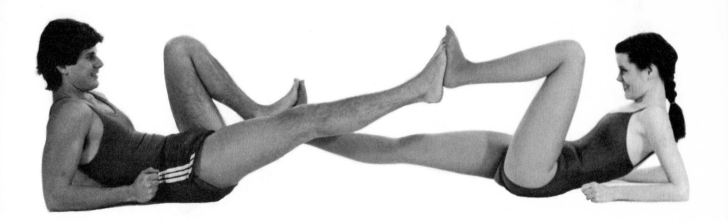

E UNDER THE BRIDGE

BENEFITS While stretching the spine and back of the legs, this exercise also firms and tones the legs, arms, and shoulders.

THE EXERCISE Stand back to back about a foot apart. Bend forward and bring your hands to the floor between your legs. Clasp each other's wrists.

One of you begin by pulling your partner's wrists toward you, then let her pull your wrists toward her, establishing a gentle seesaw motion.

Each back and forth sequence counts as 1. Do this exercise 10 times.

DOS AND DON'TS Allow your entire upper body to stretch as your partner pulls. Don't strain or rush. Exhale into the stretch; don't hold your breath.

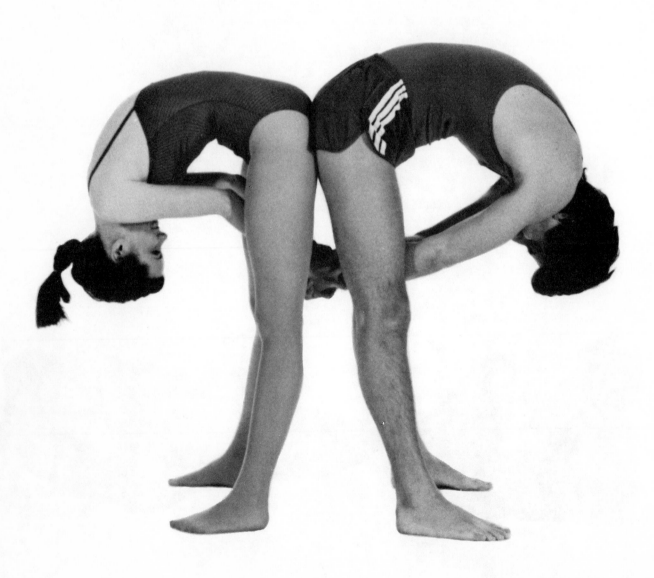

E HIGH HIP PRESS

BENEFITS This exercise strengthens the entire leg as well as firming and toning the inner thigh, buttocks, and hips.

THE EXERCISE Kneel down and place your hands on the floor in front of you. You should be parallel to each other, facing in opposite directions but with your hips next to each other. Keep your backs flat, your abdomens tight, and your heads up.

Lift your inside legs to hip height, bending the lower part of the leg back toward your buttocks. Press your thighs against each other's upraised thighs. As one of you provides resistance, the other pushes against her for a count of 10. Rest for the count of 10, then switch so the other provides resistance as the first one pushes against her.

Reverse sides and repeat with the other legs.

DOS AND DON'TS Remember to keep your elbows straight, your backs flat, your abdomens tight, and your heads up.

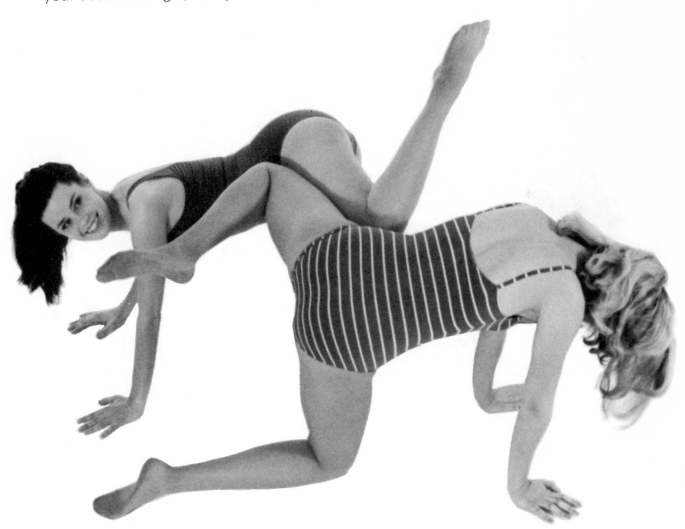

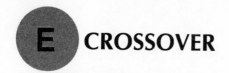

E CROSSOVER

BENEFITS This exercise builds strength in the calves, ankles, and feet, as well as firming and toning the entire leg.

THE EXERCISE Lie on your backs, heads away from each other. Prop yourselves up on your elbows and stretch your legs, feet flexed, toward each other.

One of you lift your left leg twelve inches from the floor and press on the outside of the other's raised right foot. Push inward as she provides resistance. Hold for a count of 3, then release.

Do this exercise 10 times, then 10 times with your right leg against your partner's left.

Reverse roles and repeat the entire sequence.

DOS AND DON'TS Keep your knees straight.

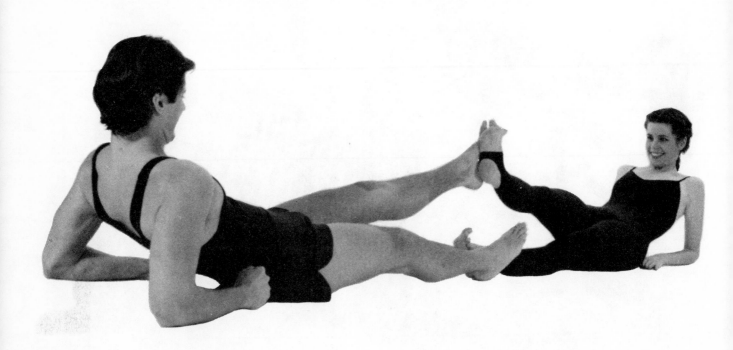

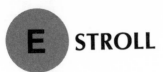 **STROLL**

BENEFITS Besides firming and toning the entire length of the legs, this exercise strengthens the legs and trims inches from the hips and buttocks.

THE EXERCISE Lie flat on your backs, heads away from each other, with your buttocks touching and your legs straight up in the air (at right angles to your bodies) and pressed against each other's. Keep your arms on the floor, but stretch them forward to hold each other's hands.

Take a walk in the air as shown. Take long strides as you each press one leg toward the other's leg while providing resistance against the leg pushing toward you.

Do this exercise 30 times back and forth with a 10-count rest between each set of 10.

DOS AND DON'TS Keep your heads, shoulders, and lower backs pressed to the floor, and your abdomens tight. Walk with a smooth, rhythmic motion. Don't hold your breath!

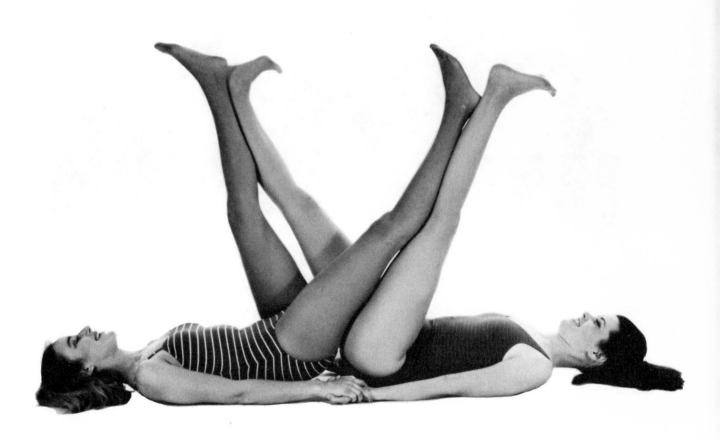

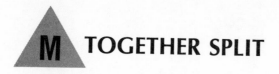 **TOGETHER SPLIT**

BENEFITS This is an excellent stretch for the inner thighs and lower backs; it also creates flexibility in the hips and pelvis.

THE EXERCISE Sit facing each other approximately six feet apart, your legs stretched open to the sides.

Bend forward and put your hands as far up each other's arms as you can. Then alternate gently pressing each other's upper body toward the floor as you relax deeper into the stretch. Hold for a count of 10 seconds, then release.

Do this exercise 3 times for each partner.

DOS AND DON'TS Remember to keep your knees straight and your feet flexed. Use relaxation and breathing to intensify your stretch, exhaling as you press toward the floor.

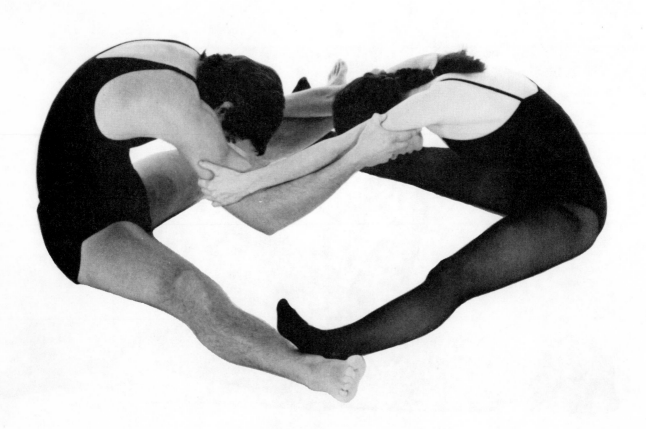

LEG LIFT WITH RESISTANCE

BENEFITS This exercise strengthens and tones the entire leg, especially calf, ankle, and foot. It also tightens and tones the inner thigh.

THE EXERCISE Lie on your sides as shown. Use the elbow of your lower arms to support your heads. To maintain your balance, press your upper hand on the floor in front of your chest.

Keeping your bodies in a straight line, but your lower legs slightly bent, one of you place your upper leg under and halfway up your partner's upper leg. Slowly lift your leg to a maximum height of twelve inches while your partner provides resistance. Release. Keep your legs straight.

Do this exercise 20 times, resting for the count of 10 between the two sets of 10. Switch leg positions with your partner and repeat.

Then roll over on your other sides and repeat the entire sequence, the lower legs now the upper.

DOS AND DON'TS Be careful not to move your hips from side to side and don't lean back on your buttocks. It's all right if you lean slightly forward.

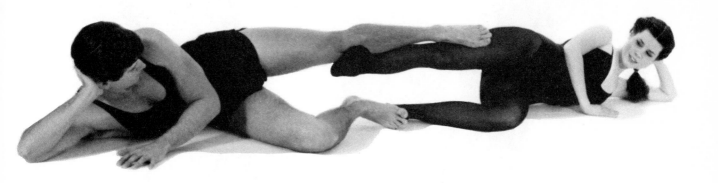

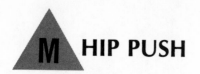 # HIP PUSH

BENEFITS Besides being a wonderful stretch for the entire side, this exercise also firms and tones the arms, hips, and legs.

THE EXERCISE Stand beside each other, about two feet apart, feet together.

Raise your arms and then reach sideways toward each other. Cross arms and grasp each other's wrists as shown, right wrist to right wrist, left to left. As you pull each other's arms toward the center, stretch your hips out to the side. Hold for a count of 10 and release.

Do this exercise 3 times, then change sides with each other and repeat.

DOS AND DON'TS Stretch your hips as far to the side as possible. Do not lean forward or backward.

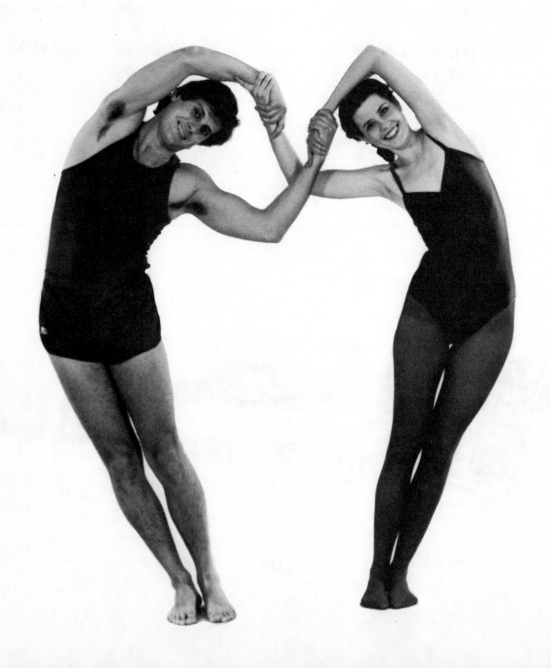

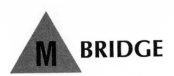 **BRIDGE**

BENEFITS Besides strengthening the legs and lower back, this exercise improves balance and coordination and provides an excellent stretch for the entire body.

THE EXERCISE Stand as if you were side by side, but four feet apart and facing each other. Stretch forward and rest your inside hands on each other's shoulders, keeping your torsos parallel to the floor.

As you do so, lift your inside legs and extend them backward so that they, too, are parallel to the floor, and stretch your outside arms forward. Your hips should be level and facing the floor. Hold for the count of 10. Now bring your legs and outer arms back to your sides.

Do this exercise 3 times, then change sides: If your left sides were the inner sides, now your right sides are. Your right legs lift back, your right arms rest on each other's shoulders.

Repeat 3 times.

DOS AND DON'TS You should both raise the same leg. Keep your abdomens tight and do the exercise smoothly and with control. Breathe normally.

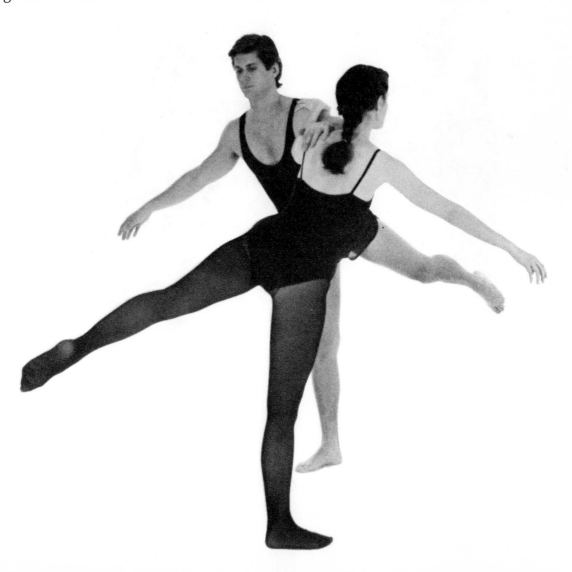

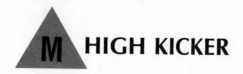 # HIGH KICKER

BENEFITS Besides providing an excellent stretch for the legs, this exercise helps improve posture, balance, and coordination. In the lifting role, the exercise also strengthens the body.

THE EXERCISE One of you kneel on your left leg in front of the other, who remains standing. As the standing partner places her left ankle on your right shoulder, clasp her right wrist while she clasps your left. Support her raised left ankle with your right hand (her left hand gently rests on that leg).

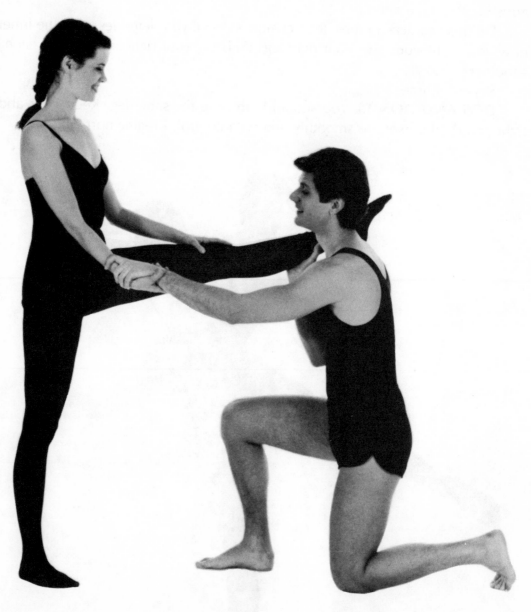

Stand up slowly and carefully, gently pushing up the leg resting on your shoulder as you do so. Then kneel slowly back down.

Do this exercise 3 times. Repeat with the other leg.

Then reverse roles and repeat the entire sequence.

DOS AND DON'TS Both partners should keep their abdomens tight and backs straight. Do this exercise carefully, with as much control as possible. Breathe normally; holding your breath will *not* help you maintain your balance.

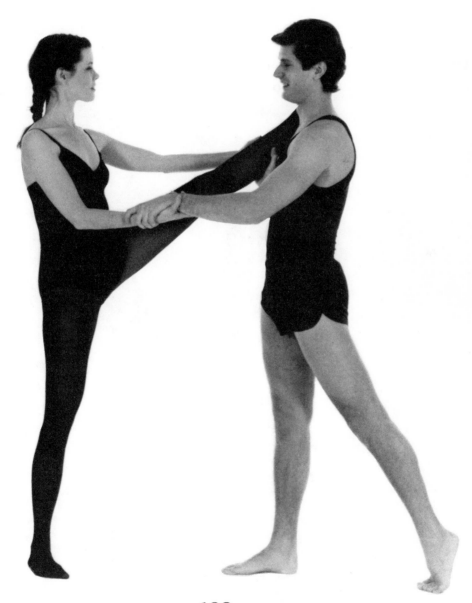

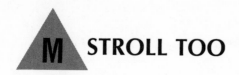

▲M STROLL TOO

BENEFITS Besides firming and toning the entire length of the legs, this exercise strengthens the legs and trims inches from the hips and buttocks. It also strengthens and tones the abdomen.

THE EXERCISE Lie flat on your backs, heads away from each other, with your buttocks touching and your legs straight up in the air (at right angles to your bodies) and pressed against each other's. Lift your heads and shoulders from the floor as you reach forward and grab each other's hands.

Take a walk with your legs in the air, as shown. Take long strides as you each press one leg toward the other's leg while providing resistance against the leg pushing toward you.

Do this exercise 30 times back and forth with a 10-count rest between each set of 10.

DOS AND DON'TS Keep your heads and shoulders up from the floor and your abdomens tight. Walk with a smooth, rhythmic motion. Don't hold your breath!

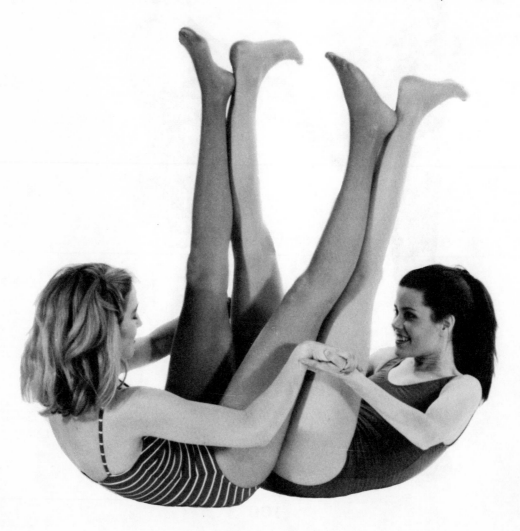

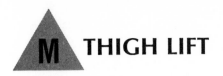# M THIGH LIFT

BENEFITS This exercise is a wonderful stretch for the front of the thighs, hips, abdomens, shoulders, and arms. In the lifting role, the exercise also helps develop strength and endurance.

THE EXERCISE One of you stand with your back to the other, who is kneeling on her outward rotated right leg and has her left one bent, as shown. Lift your right leg backward and place it on her right shoulder. As you do so, your right hand and her left one should clasp each other's wrist. Lean forward, keeping a tight grip on your partner's wrist while she slowly stands up, stretching your leg as she does so, and then returns to her original kneeling position.

Do this exercise 3 times, then change legs, shoulders, and arms and repeat.

Finally, reverse roles and repeat the entire sequence.

DOS AND DON'TS Be sure not to strain. Do this exercise with as much control as possible. Whether you are lifting or stretching, keep your abdomen tight. Don't hold your breath.

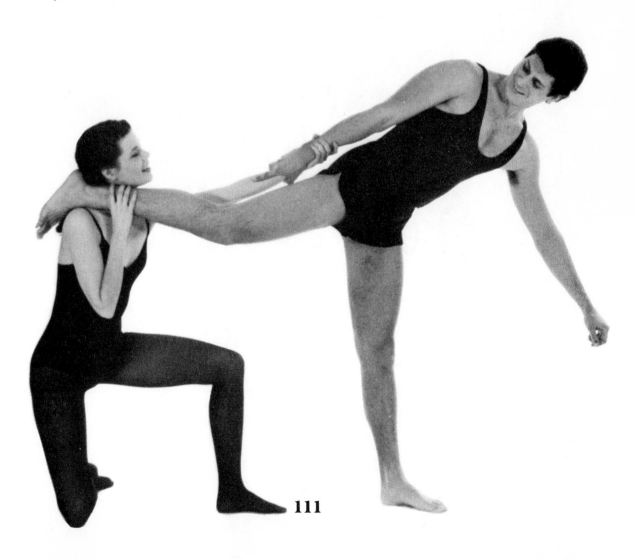

111

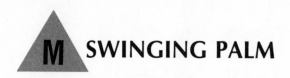 **SWINGING PALM**

BENEFITS This exercise stretches and strengthens the leg muscles, opens the chest and shoulders, and relieves tension throughout the spine.

THE EXERCISE Stand facing each other, about a foot away and spread your legs about two feet apart. Turn your front feet forward and your back feet in, as shown. Extend your arms out to the side at shoulder level and clasp each other's hands.

Turn toward your front legs and bring your front arms down to the floor while your rear arms swing over your heads toward the ceiling.

Hold for a count of 10 and return to the upright position.

Do this exercise 3 times, then reposition your feet and turn in the other direction so you repeat on the other side.

DOS AND DON'TS Be sure to do the movements slowly and evenly. Keep your arms straight. Exhale into the stretch; inhale as you come up.

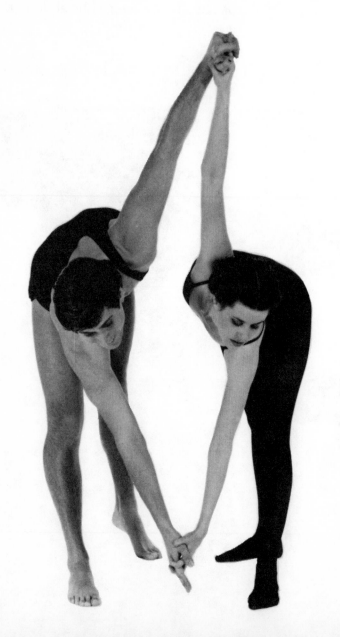

H TWISTING T

BENEFITS Besides being a terrific stretch for the entire body, this exercise also firms and tones the legs, hips, and arms.

THE EXERCISE Stand back to back, arms stretched out in a **T**. One of you clasp the other's wrist.

Both of you bend over to the other side, lifting the clasped arms straight up in the air. Place the fingers of your free arms onto the floor and twist your heads to look up at the raised arms. Turn your front feet forward, as shown, and bend the front knees to lower your bodies as far down as you can.

Return to starting position. Switch sides and repeat, stretching and bending in the other direction.

DOS AND DON'TS Remember to turn your heads to look at your raised arms. Keep your bodies straight; don't lean forward or back. Keep your abdomens tight.

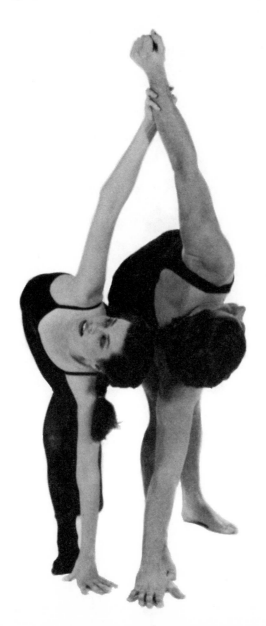

H   TOE-DOWN LIFT

BENEFITS This exercise firms and tones the thighs as well as strengthening the entire leg, buttocks, and abdomen.

THE EXERCISE Lie on your sides facing each other. Each of you rest your head on one hand and place the other in front of you for balance.

Each of you bend your bottom leg slightly, then lift your top leg about twelve inches and extend it forward to meet your partner's foot. One of you place your foot over your partner's with your toe pointed down and your heel up. As he pushes his foot up, you provide resistance.

Reverse foot positions so you push and he resists.

Do this exercise 30 times in each position, resting for a count of 10 between each set of 10.

Then change sides so the bottom leg is now the top and repeat the entire sequence, reversing roles after 30 times.

DOS AND DON'TS Keep the upper legs lifted straight out from the hips, and don't bend the knees or allow the legs to drop. Remember that the lower legs should stay bent. Breathe normally.

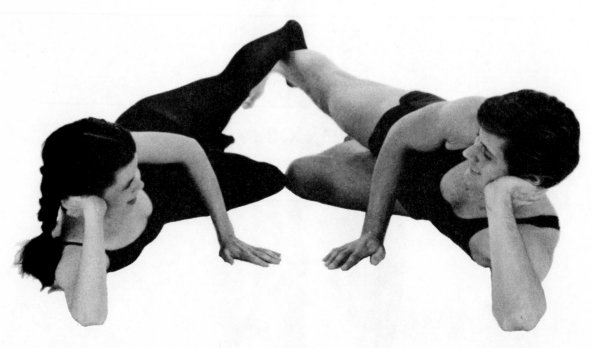

H SPLIT LIFT

BENEFITS This exercise is a wonderful stretch for the inner thigh. In the lifting role, the exercise builds up the body's strength and endurance.

THE EXERCISE Stand sideways in front of your partner, who is kneeling on one leg. Twist your upper body toward her and clasp her left wrist with your right hand. Lift your left leg onto her right shoulder, making sure your knee is rotated inward. Then keep a firm grip on her wrist as she slowly stands up, stretching your leg, and then kneels down again.

Do this exercise 3 times, then change directions so your right leg rests on her left shoulder and repeat. Reverse roles and repeat the entire sequence.

DOS AND DON'TS The partner who is being lifted should keep his abdomen tight and be sure that his knee is rotated inward. Do this exercise with control; don't rush.

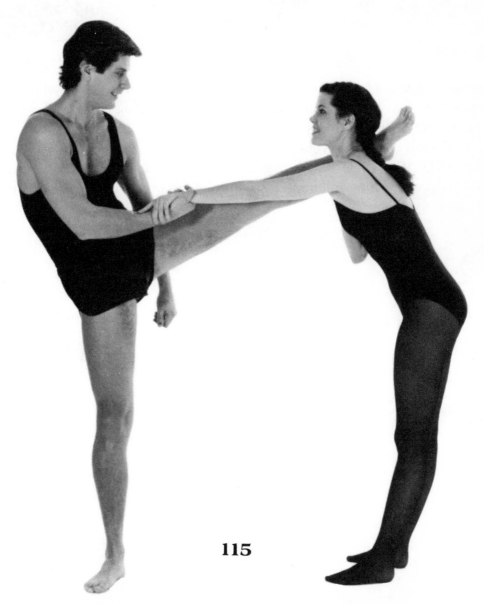

H SWAN

BENEFITS This exercise firms and tones the entire thigh while toning the hips and buttocks. In addition, it provides an excellent stretch for the front of the torso.

THE EXERCISE Lie on your sides, back to back, about a foot apart and with both arms above your heads. Rest your heads on the lower arm. Bend both arms back toward each other and grasp each other's right wrists with right hands, left wrists with left hands.

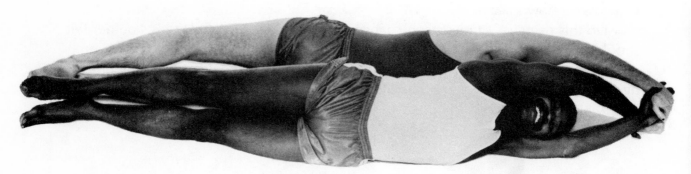

Extend your arms back toward each other and lift them. At the same time, press your lower hips into the floor and lift your top legs, bringing them backward to push against each other's leg and foot for a count of 10.

Change sides, reassume your positions, and repeat.

DOS AND DON'TS Extend throughout your arms and legs and press your pelvises forward. Try not to strain, and don't rush through the exercise. Exhale as you lift your leg; inhale as you release.

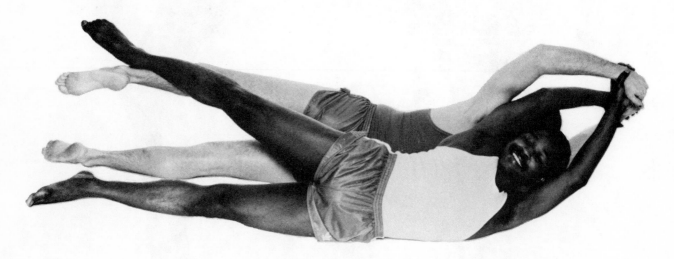

116

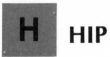 HIP LIFT WITH FRIEND

BENEFITS This exercise strengthens the entire leg and tightens and firms the buttock muscles.

THE EXERCISE Lie on your stomachs side by side, hands under your chins, elbows out to the side.

Reach forward with your outside arms and lift your upper bodies off the floor, supporting the weight on your inside elbows, as shown. With your legs stretched out straight behind you, raise the outside legs from your hip and swing them toward each other, crossing them at the ankles. The leg on top pushes down toward the floor as the leg below provides resistance. Hold for a count of 10, then release. Switch positions so the other partner's leg is on top and repeat.

Then switch sides so the inner legs are now the outer, and repeat this entire sequence.

DOS AND DON'TS Allow only the hips of the outer legs to lift while doing the exercise; keep the inner hips pressed firmly into the floor. Don't force the exercise.

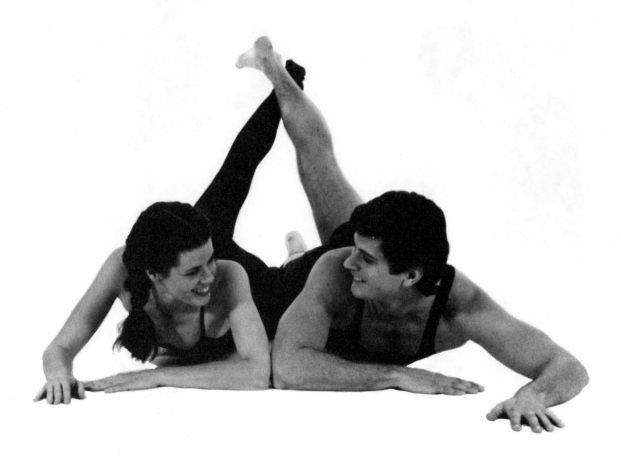

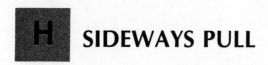

H SIDEWAYS PULL

BENEFITS This exercise is a vigorous stretch for the entire side of the body, and also firms and tones the arms, hips, and legs.

THE EXERCISE Stand side by side, but two to three feet apart. Keeping your feet together, extend your arms upward and over toward each other and clasp hands as shown, right hand to right, left hand to left.

Stretch your hips and entire torsos to the outer side, extending your arms as far as you can, so that your entire weight is pulling against each other's. Hold for the count of 10. Release.

Switch sides and repeat.

DOS AND DON'TS Stretch your arms as well as your torsos. Keep your heads aligned with the rest of your bodies, and be careful not to lean either forward or back. Breathe normally. If you exhale for the stretch, you will achieve greater flexibility.

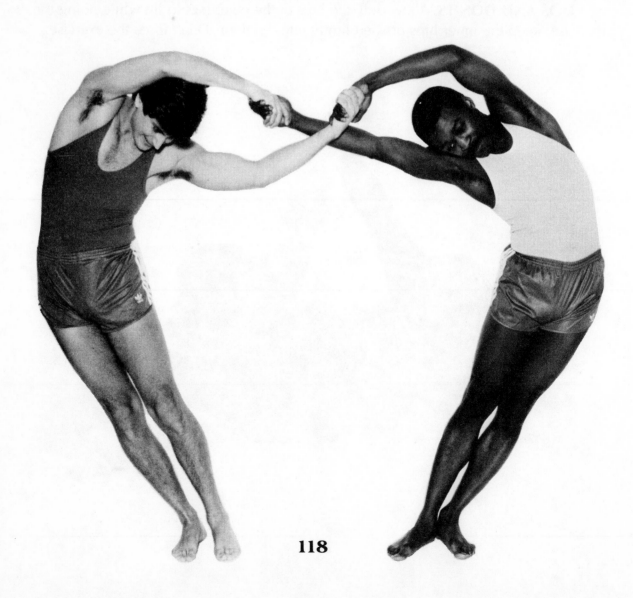

118

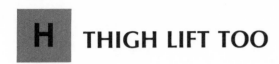

H THIGH LIFT TOO

BENEFITS This exercise is a wonderful stretch for the front of the thighs, as well as the hips, abdomen, shoulders, and arms. In the lifting role, the exercise helps develop strength and endurance.

THE EXERCISE One of you stand with your back to the other, who is kneeling on his outward rotated right leg and has his left one bent. Lift your right leg backward and place it on his right shoulder. As you do so, your right hand and his left one should clasp each other's wrist. Lean forward, keeping a tight grip on your partner's wrist while he slowly stands up, stretching your leg as he does so, then returns to his original kneeling position.

Do this exercise 6 times, then change legs, shoulders, and arms and repeat.

Finally, reverse roles and repeat the entire sequence.

DOS AND DON'TS Be sure not to strain. Do this exercise with as much control as possible. Whether you are lifting or stretching, keep your abdomen tight. Don't hold your breath.

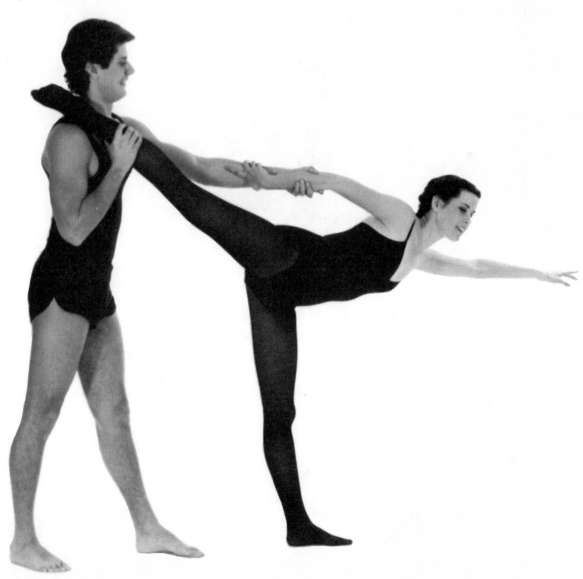

H HIKE

BENEFITS This is an excellent exercise for strengthening the legs and lower back, and it also serves as a toner for the abdomen and buttocks.

THE EXERCISE Lie flat on your backs, heads away from each other, with your buttocks touching and your legs straight up in the air (at right angles to your bodies) and lightly pressed against each other's. Your feet should be flexed.

Lift your heads and shoulders from the floor and extend your arms forward, keeping them parallel to the floor, as shown. Keep your legs, buttocks, and abdomens tight and press your lower backs into the floor.

Take a walk with your legs in the air. Take long strides as you each press one leg toward the other's leg while providing resistance against the leg pushing toward you.

Do this exercise 30 times back and forth with a 10-count rest between each set of 10.

DOS AND DON'TS If you feel you're losing control, hold onto your partner's wrists. Don't rush the exercise, and don't hold your breath.

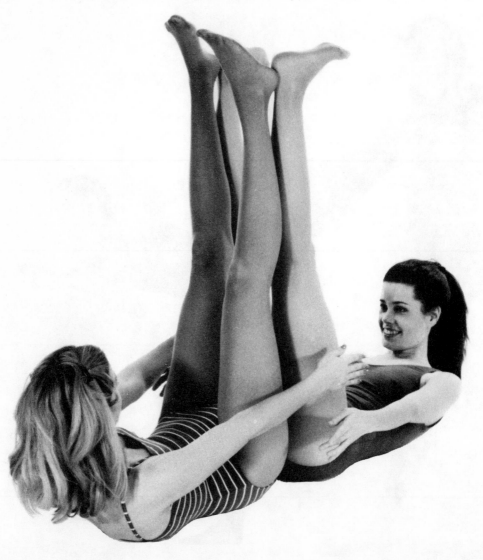

E. cardiovascular exercises

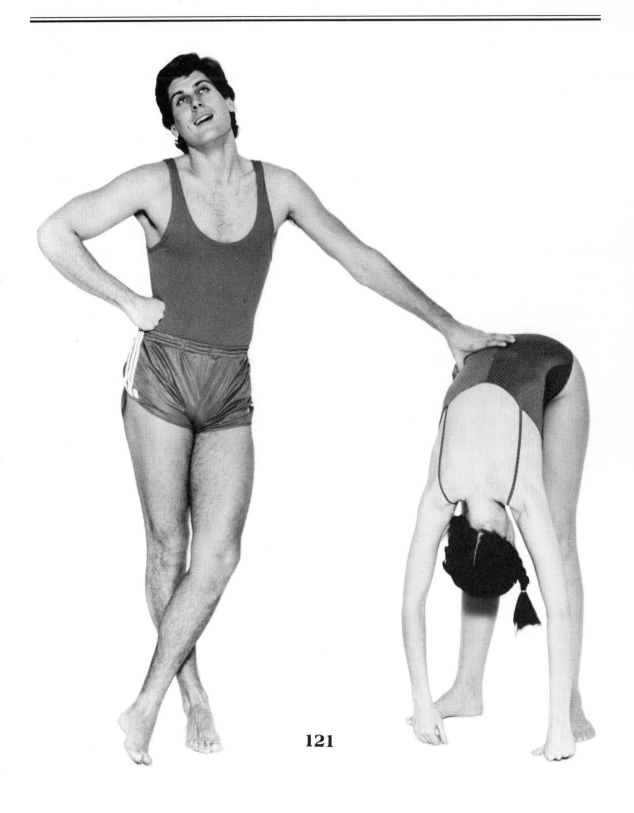

*B*ESIDES KEEPING your bodies fit, it's important to keep your hearts fit. After all, the heart *is* the most important muscle in the body!

The cardiovascular exercise program that follows is an integral part of the couples' fitness program. It provides the physical workout your hearts need to get and stay strong and healthy.

Inactivity and stress are two of the major factors implicated in heart conditions that can actually be helped by exercise. Studies show that the death rate from heart attacks among sedentary people is more than twice as great as among physically active individuals. Frequently heart problems start when the heart muscle becomes weak and can no longer pump an adequate volume of blood to the lungs and the rest of the body.

As for stress—well, by now stress is infamous as a major component in heart problems. Some researchers believe that a specific personality type is particularly susceptible to heart disease and to other stress-related ailments. This is the so-called Type-A personality: hard driving, a compulsive worker, one who tends to suppress fatigue and attempts to control everything and everyone around him or her. This personality type is constantly fighting anxiety, frustration, and worry—not always successfully! But no matter what the personality type, in today's fast-moving electronic/computer/space-age world, *all* of us suffer from various degrees of stress.

Exercise eliminates inactivity and reduces stress. These exercises in particular work not only to strengthen the heart and lungs, but they also build strength and endurance in the entire body. The benefits are many: lower blood pressure, increased blood output per heart beat, increased blood oxygen, greater breathing efficiency, reduced blood cholesterol, increased muscle flexibility and tone, increased stamina and, last but hardly least, a wonderful, *relaxed* feeling.

So go to it!

As you undertake this program, do so carefully. Pay attention to your pulse rate and breathing. The physical exam your doctor gives you before you start the couples' exercise program should, of course, include a cardiovascular stress test so that you have a clear picture of your current state of cardiovascular fitness before you start.

Although there is a continuing controversy in medical circles over just what the maximally beneficial pulse rate during exercise should be, and many complex formulas have been suggested, a simple formula—and one that works—is to subtract your age from 170. This will give you your optimum heart rate.

To check what your heart rate is, stop the cardiovascular exercise after five minutes, take your pulse for fifteen seconds and multiply by four.

If the answer is below your recommended optimum rate, continue exercising. If your pulse is faster than your optimum, stop. The next day, exercise for only one minute and check again. Exercise a little longer each day. You should eventually be able to do the cardiovascular exercises for twelve to fifteen minutes and maintain a pulse rate that is below your maximum.

Unlike the other exercises in this program, which should be done slowly and carefully, the idea behind the cardiovascular series of exercises is to keep up a steady demand on the body, heart, and lungs to make the session aeorobically challenging.

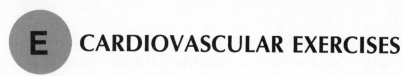 **E** **CARDIOVASCULAR EXERCISES**

Do all these exercises in sequence without stopping between each.

   1. Jog in place without lifting your feet off the floor. The motion is heel, toe, heel, toe. Do for a count of 20: 1-heel, 2-toe.
   2. Keep jogging in place, but now bring your feet off the floor and your knees waist high for a count of 20: 1-left, 2-right.
   3. Prance, bringing your knees as high as you can for a count of 20: 1-left, 2-right.

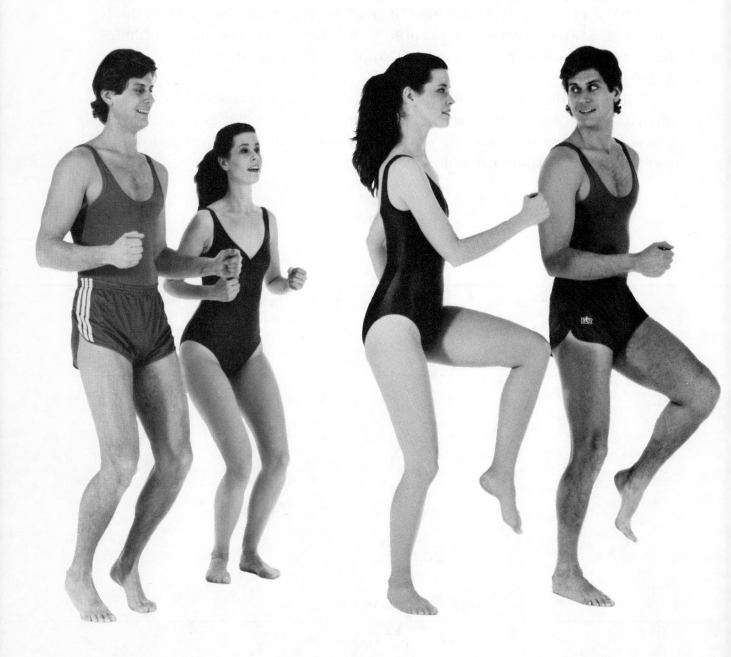

4. Jump and twist your bodies to the left at the same time as you bring your arms over to the right, as shown. Then jump and twist to the right, at the same time as you bring your arms over to the left. Do this for a count of 20: 1-left, 2-right.

5. Reverse the jogging sequence, beginning with the prance, for a count of 20.

6. Jog in place, bringing your knees waist high for a count of 20.

7. Do the heel/toe jog (without lifting your foot from the floor) for a count of 20.

8. Jump and twist your bodies to the right at the same time as you bring your arms over to the left. Then jump and twist left, bringing your arms right. Do for a count of 20.

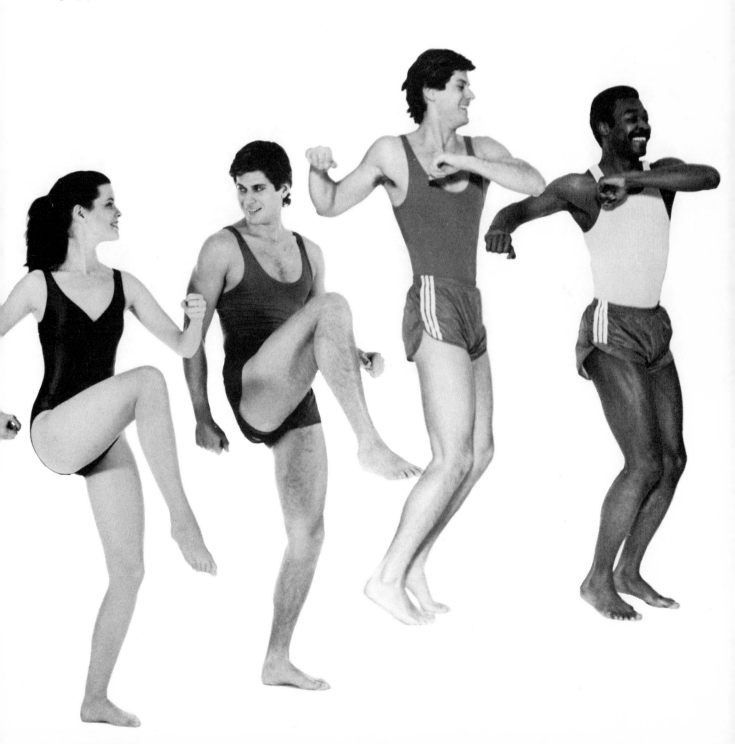

9. With your feet together, hop forward and to the right, then jump back; hop forward and to the left. Repeat this sequence for a count of 20.

10. Hop up and down. Count when your feet touch down and do for a count of 20.

11. Repeat the hopping exercise (number 9) for a count of 20.

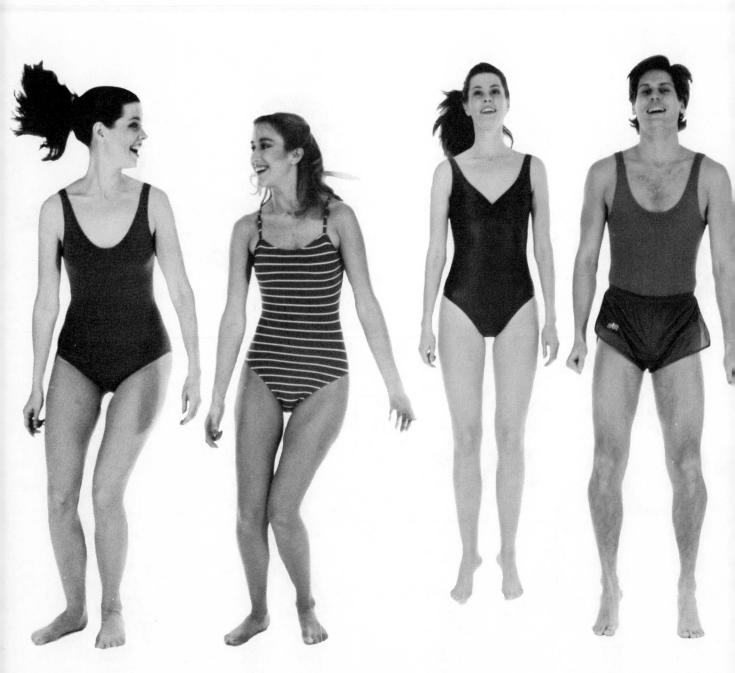

12. Do jumping jacks by jumping in the air and opening your legs, landing with your legs apart at the same time as you swing your arms up over your head to clap your hands. Return by jumping up and landing with your feet together, bringing your arms down to your sides. Do this sequence to a count of 20 jumping jacks in all.

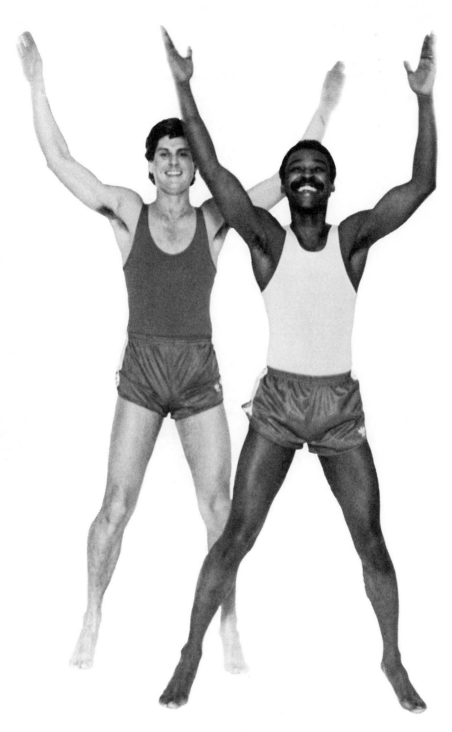

13. Bend over to your ankles and start to cross your arms at the wrists. Keep crossing and recrossing while you roll your body back up and bring your arms over your head. Keep a heel/toe jog (see exercise 1) going while you are doing this. Do to a count of 20.

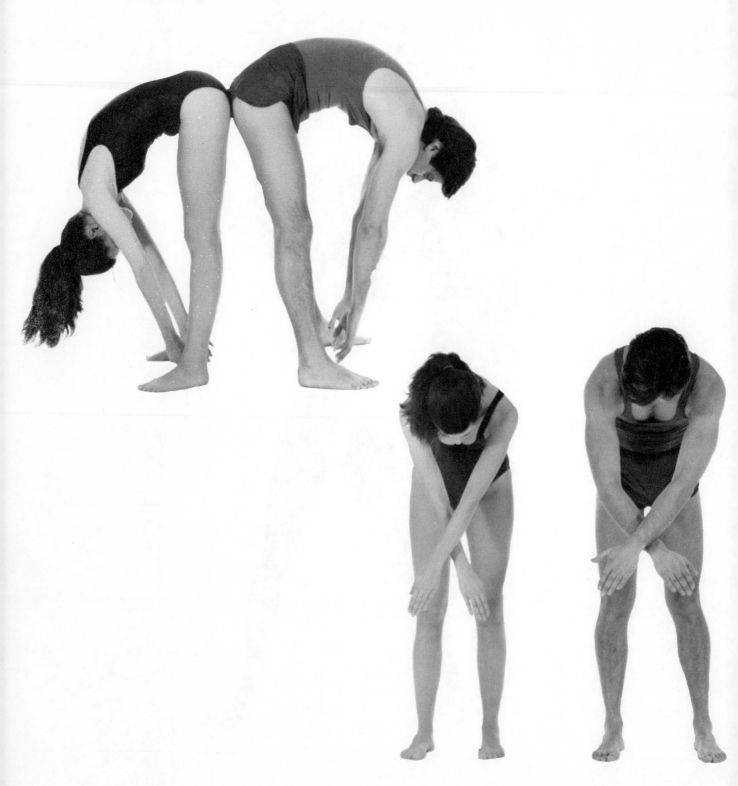

14. Continue a heel/toe jog while you cross and uncross your arms at chest level for a count of 20.

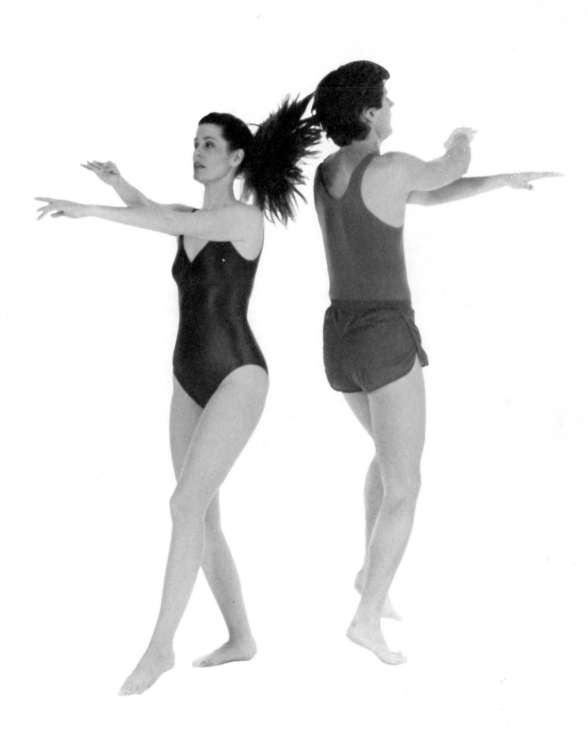

15. Bend forward and swing your arms between your legs, then come forward into a flat-back position, swinging your arms straight out in front of you. The sequence of back and forward is 1 count. Do for a count of 20.

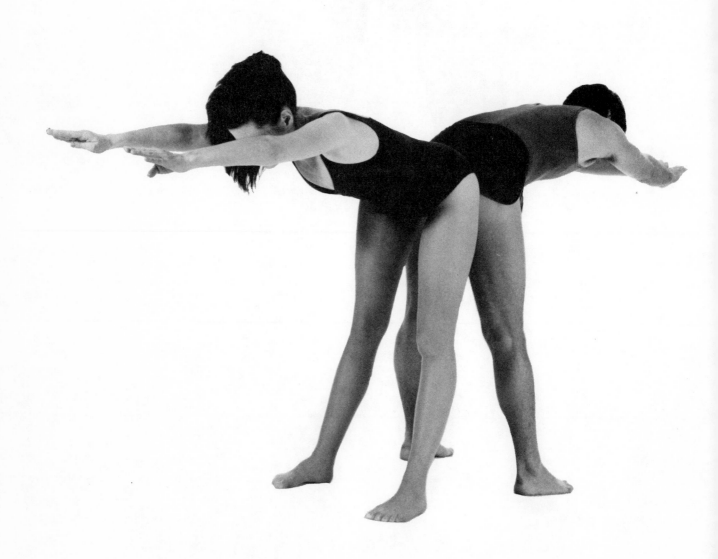

16. From the flat-back position, bring one arm down to the floor while bringing the other one up in the air. Twist your head and upper body to look at the overhead arm. Return to flat-back position. Repeat with the other arm. Do for a count of 20: 1-left, 2-right.

17. Jog in place without lifting your feet off the floor, as in exercise 1, for a count of 20.

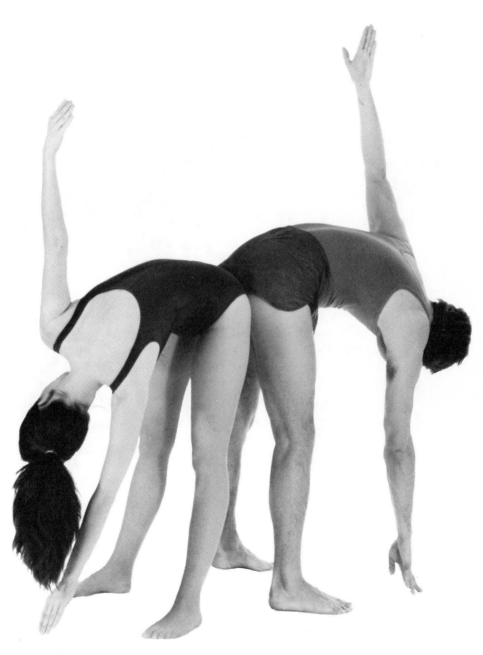

18. Take a deep breath and bend forward, exhaling into the stretch. Grasp your ankles with your hands and gently stretch your body toward your legs. Hold, breathing deeply, for a count of 10.

19. Bend your knees and lower your body to the floor.

Relax.

Congratulations!

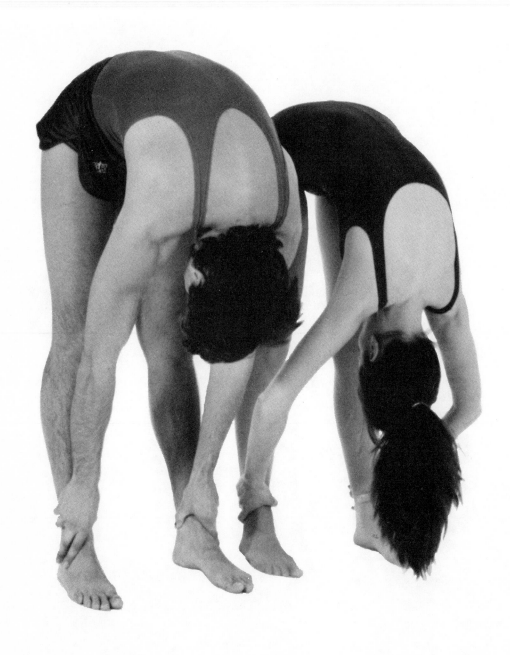

CARDIOVASCULAR EXERCISES

Do all these exercises in sequence without stopping between each.

    1. Skip in place, for 1 minute.
    2. Hop on one leg, holding the other leg up behind you, for 1 minute. Change legs and hop for 1 minute.

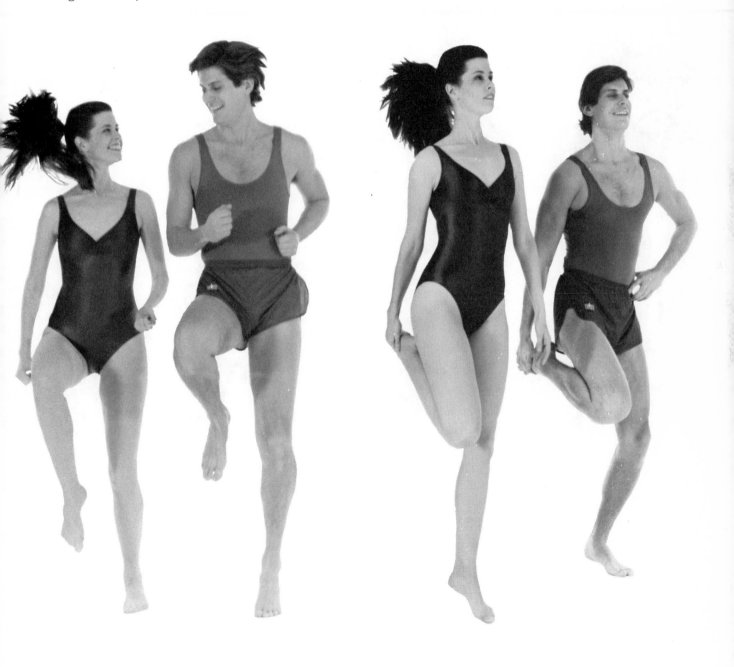

3. Hop on one foot with your other foot out, as shown, for 1 minute. Change legs and hop for 1 minute.

4. Jog in place, shifting from heel to toe without lifting your feet. Hold your arms up over your head and stretch and reach first with your right arm, then with your left. Do this exercise for a count of 10: 1-right, 2-left.

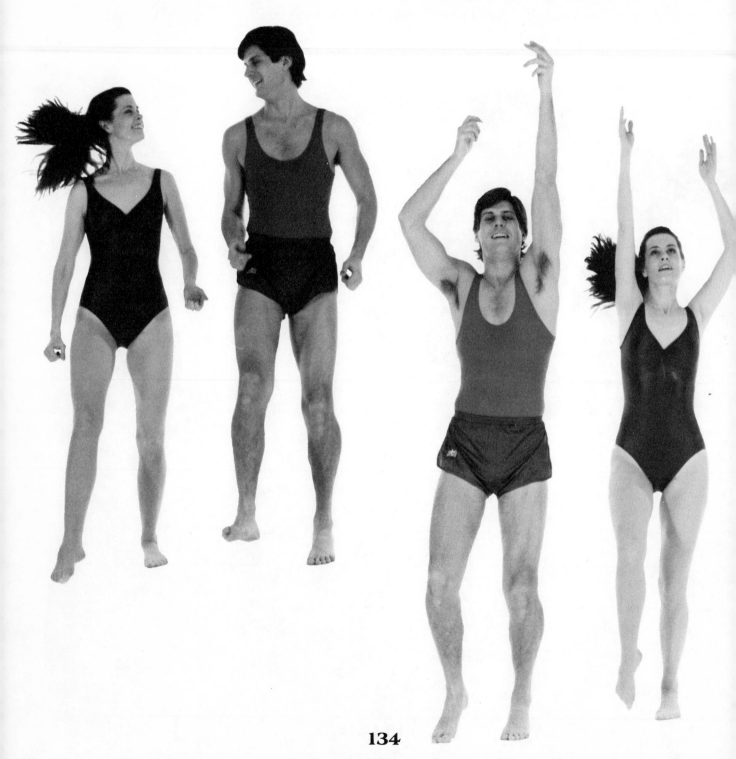

5. Hop in place while circling with your outstretched arms for a count of 20.

6. Jump up as you twist your arms to the right, then to the left. Do this exercise for a count of 20: 1-right, 2-left.

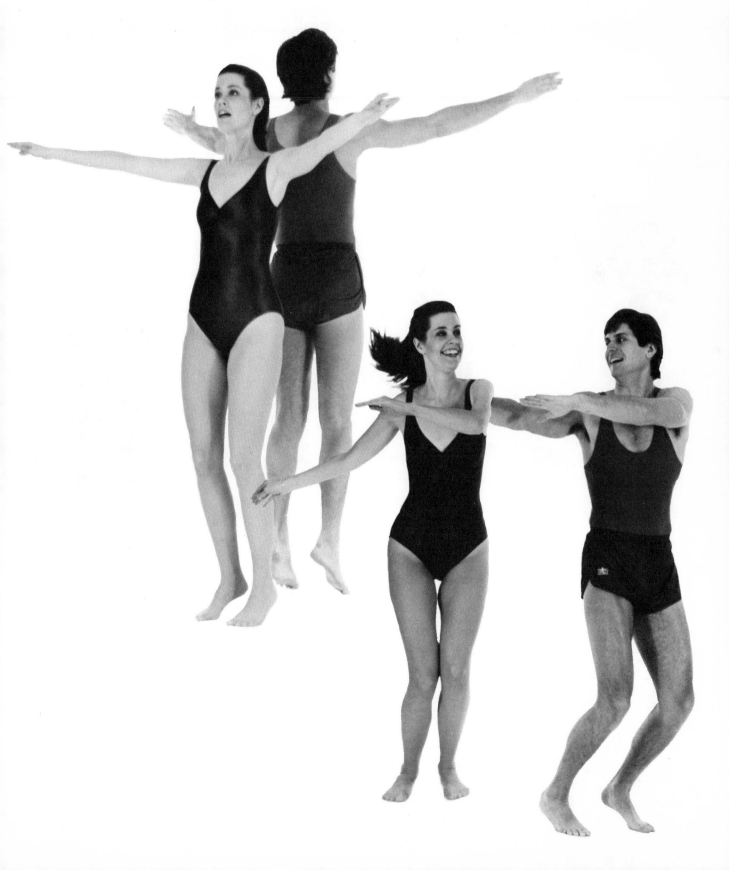

7. Bend forward and reach down with one arm while pulling your other arm up as high as you can, elbow leading, as if you were pulling weeds. Alternate arms for a count of 20, each arm counting as 1.

8. Skip, keeping your knees high and lifting your arms toward the ceiling. Stretch and reach with one arm, then with the other. Do this exercise for a count of 20, each arm counting as 1.

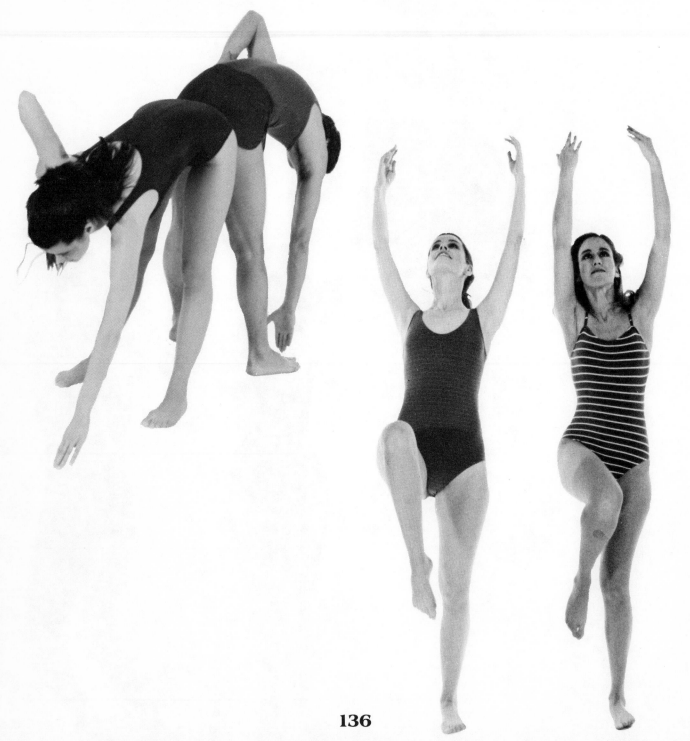

9. Lean forward to a flat-back position, swing your arms back behind you, and then swing them down to the floor. Do this exercise for a count of 20: 1-back, 2-down.

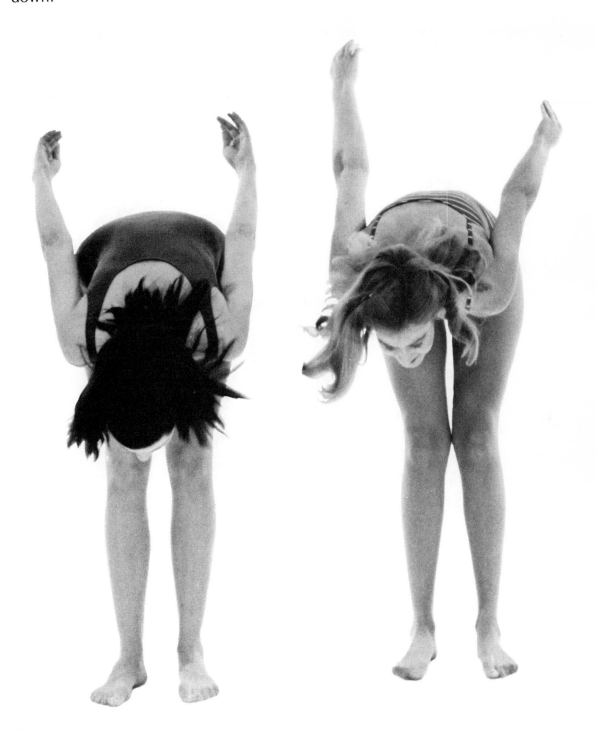

10. Stand back to back, legs open about a foot, buttocks touching. Swing your arms forward and then down through your legs toward each other's hands. Do this exercise for a count of 20: 1-forward, 2-down.

For the next sequence, use a jump rope if one is available.

11. Skip rope for 1 minute. Hop for 1 minute. Skip for 1 minute.

12. Repeat exercise 6 for a count of 20.

13. Do the heel/toe jog (your feet don't leave the floor) for a count of 20.
Relax.
Congratulations!

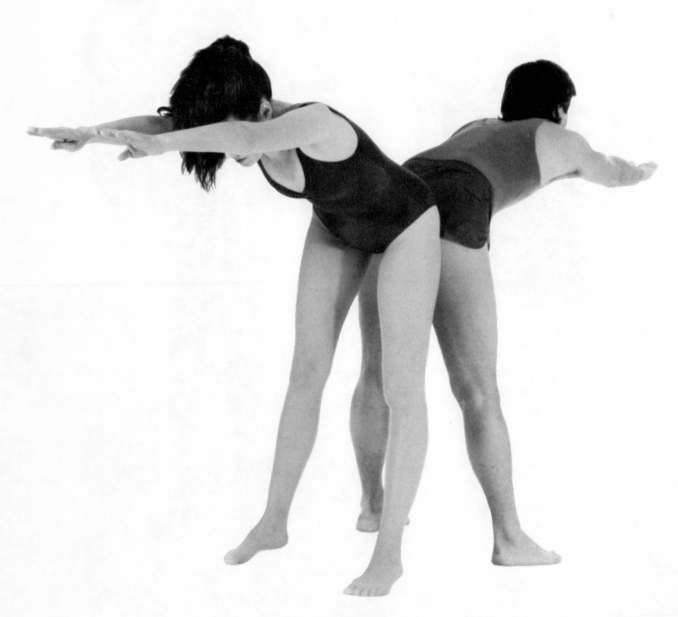

CARDIOVASCULAR EXERCISES

Do all these exercises in sequence without stopping between each.

1. Jog in place without lifting your feet off the floor. The motion is heel, toe, heel, toe, each counting 1. Do for a count of 20.

2. Jog in place with your knees higher, and lift your feet off the floor. Do for a count of 20: 1-left, 2-right.

3. Jog, pulling your knees even higher and slapping them with your hands. Do for a count of 20: 1-left, 2-right.

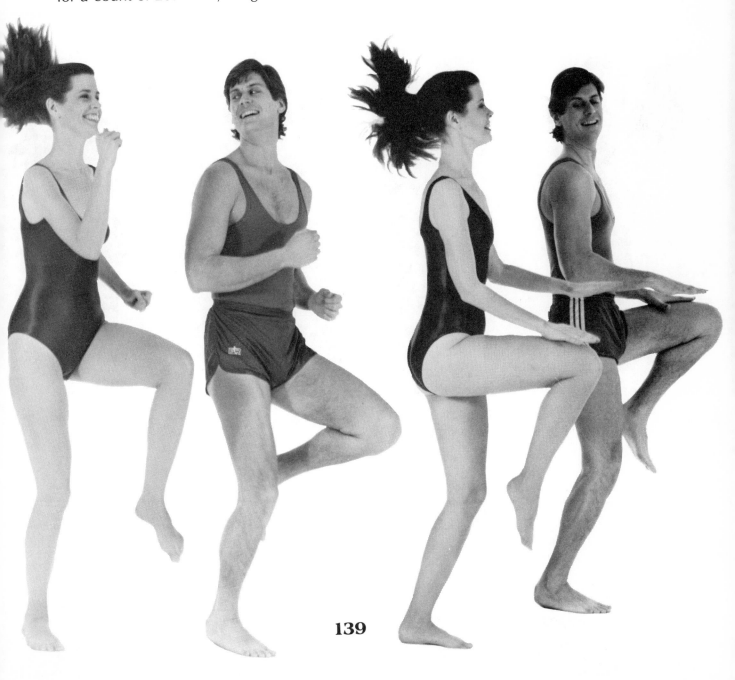

139

4. Repeat the heel/toe jog of exercise 1 and alternately stretch one arm up and the other arm down as you do so. Do for a count of 20: 1-left up, 2-right up.

5. Hop on your right foot and swing your right arm down while you swing your left leg out to the side and your left arm up. Then hop onto your left foot, left arm down, right leg out and right arm up. Do this exercise for a count of 10: 1-left, 2-right.

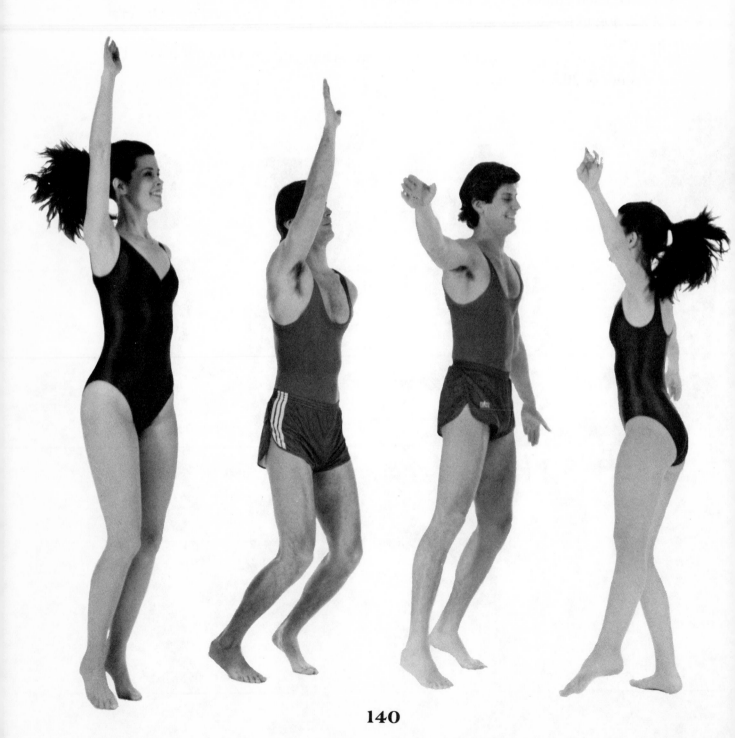

6. Hop on both feet as you cross and recross your hands overhead. Do for a count of 20: 1-hop/cross, 2-hop/cross.

7. Hop on your right foot while you swing your left leg out to the side, as in exercise 5, but now lift your left arm higher and kick your left leg higher. Alternate right and left for a count of 10.

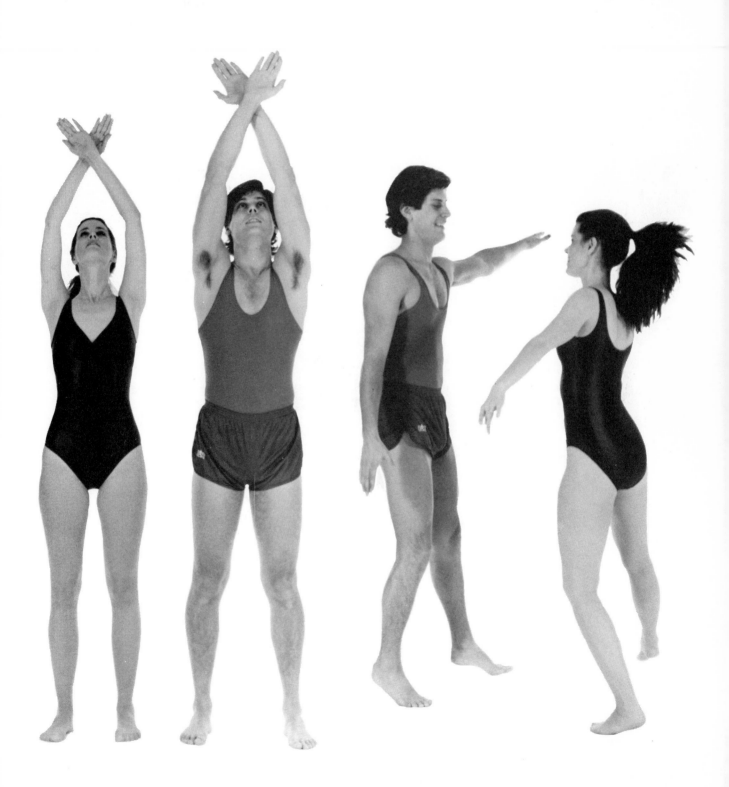

8. Lift your right knee and hip out to the right. Then hop to the right on your left foot. Step onto your right foot, then lift your left knee and hip out to the left, and hop to the left on your right foot. (This movement is much like the "Mashed Potatoes" step danced around 1960.) Do for a count of 20: 1-hop right, 2-hop left.

9. Lift your right leg behind you and then swing it straight out in front of you while hopping on your left foot. Then jump onto your right foot and swing your left leg back and then forward while hopping on your right foot. Do this exercise for a count of 20: 1-back right, 2-forward right, 3-back left, 4-forward left.

10. With your feet together, jump forward and to the right. Jump back. Then jump forward and to your left. Jump back. Repeat this sequence for a count of 10.

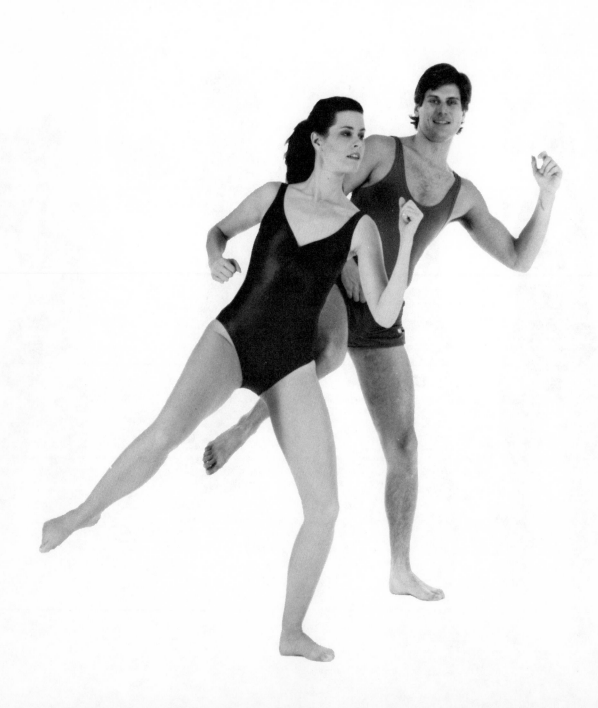

11. Repeat exercise 9 for a count of 20.

12. With your feet together, jump forward. Jump back. Then jump forward again. Do this exercise for a count of 10: 1-forward, 2-back.

13. Skip with or without a jump rope for 1 minute. Hop for 1 minute. Skip for 1 minute.

Relax.

Congratulations!

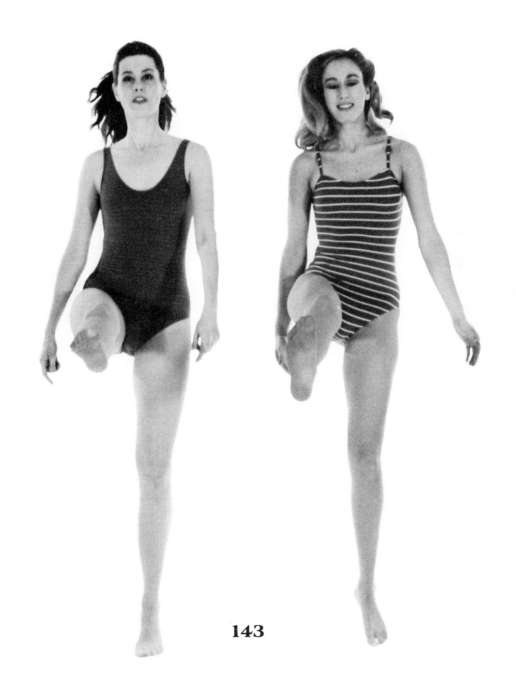

F. the cool-down

Plow

Knee-to-Ear Stretch

Easy Forward Thigh Stretch

Shoulder Stand

Easy Thigh Stretch

Knee Hold

Forward Stretch

Knee-in

Full Body Stretch

Alternate Side Stretch

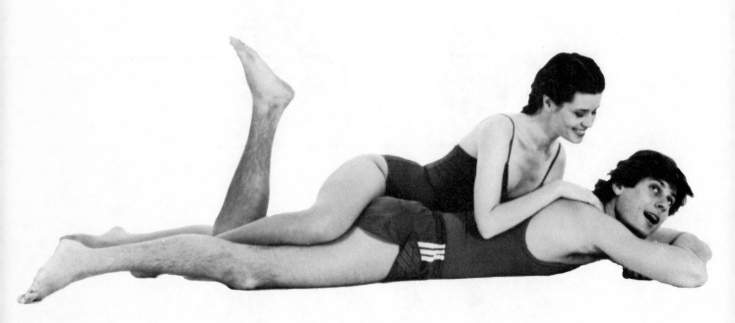

HOLD IT RIGHT THERE! YOU MAY *NOT* SKIP THE COOL-DOWN! I know you're probably tired from exercising, but if you omit this section in favor of a shower, I guarantee you'll be sorry. You'll almost certainly suffer aches and pains tomorrow; after all, 90 percent of all stiffness and pain after exercise is caused by failure to cool down.

As I told you in chapter 3, lactic acid builds up in your muscle fibers during vigorous exercise. If it remains there, soreness and cramping can be the unpleasant result. The purpose of the cool-down is to dissipate this lactic acid, (although it's a marvelous way to relax yourself as well!)

No self-respecting equestrian would dream of returning a horse to the stall after a workout without first walking him to allow him to cool down. Surely your body deserves equal treatment!

PLOW

BENEFITS This exercise releases tension, stretches the legs and back, and improves circulation.

THE EXERCISE Lie on your backs, arms at your sides.

Lift your legs up and over your bodies and rest your toes on the floor behind your heads. Hold for one to two minutes while you breathe deeply.

Pull your knees down toward your faces and, rolling down along your spines, return to your original position.

DOS AND DON'TS When your legs are behind your heads, you can if necessary support your backs with your hands. Relax and do the exercise with control.

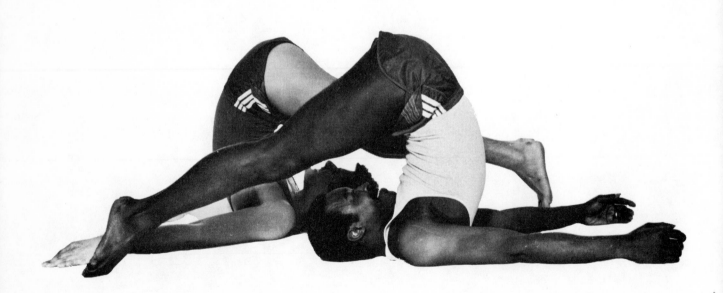

KNEE-TO-EAR STRETCH

BENEFITS This exercise streamlines and strengthens the back, spine, and legs. It also releases tension.

THE EXERCISE Lie on your backs, arms at your sides.

Pull your knees into your chests and, supporting your lower backs with your hands, swing your legs up behind your heads and onto the floor, as shown. Move your hands to lightly clasp your ankles and relax your knees in toward your ears. Hold for one to two minutes, breathing deeply.

To return to the starting position, relax your knees in toward your faces, and return your arms to your sides, pressing them against the floor. Starting at your shoulders, roll down carefully along your spines, keeping your abdomens contracted. When the full length of your spines are on the floor, relax your knees into your chests, and carefully place your feet on the floor.

DOS AND DON'TS Relax the knees in toward the ears only as far as they can go comfortably. Don't strain.

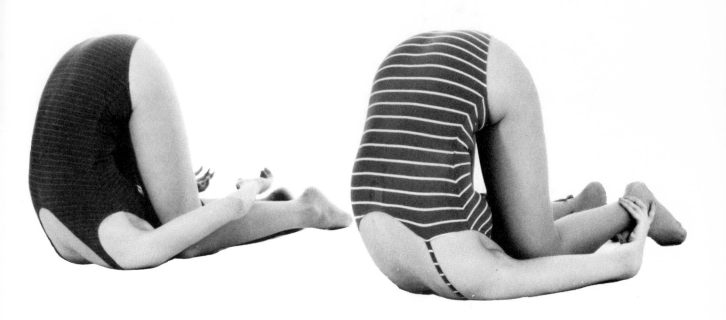

EASY FORWARD THIGH STRETCH

BENEFITS Besides stretching the thighs, knees, and legs, this exercise also releases tension throughout the spine.

THE EXERCISE Sit on the floor, bend your knees, and press the soles of your feet together. Tilt your heads back and place your hands on your knees.

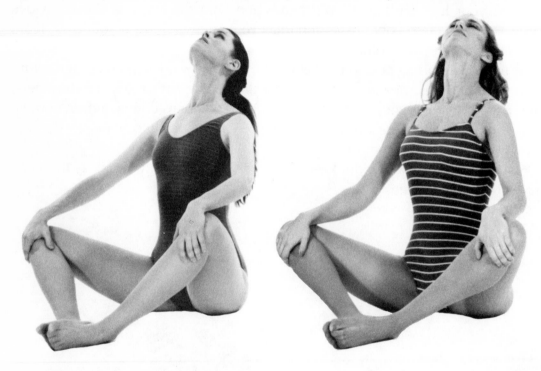

Press down on your knees with your hands and move your upper bodies forward and down, bringing your heads as close to the floor as possible. Slide your hands down to your ankles and hold your position for a count of 10. Return to the starting position.

Do this exercise 3 times.

DOS AND DON'TS Exhale as you fold forward, breathe normally while you hold, and inhale as you come up. Do the exercise with an easy, relaxed motion.

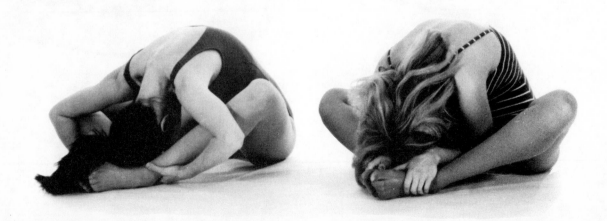

SHOULDER STAND

BENEFITS This exercise releases tension, improves circulation and body alignment, and promotes a tranquil feeling.

THE EXERCISE Lie on your backs, arms at your sides. Lift up your legs and bring your knees back toward your foreheads while you support your lower backs with your hands.

Then raise your legs, toes pointed, straight up toward the ceiling, making both your backs and legs as straight as you can.

Hold for two to three minutes.

DOS AND DON'TS Do this exercise with control: Keep your abdomens tight and breathe deeply. Don't hold your breath. Tuck your chins to your chests to avoid neck strain.

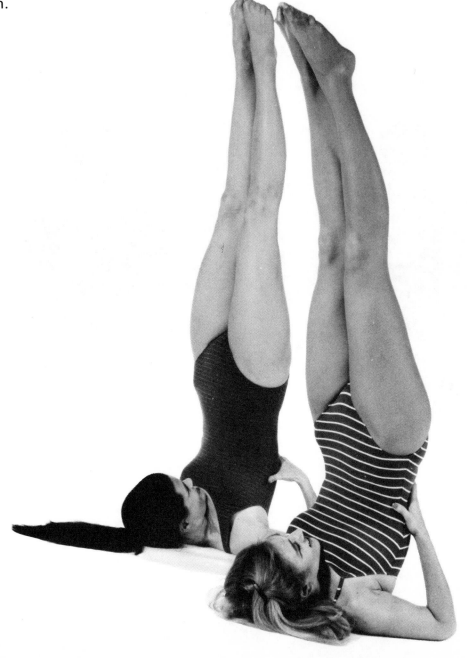

EASY THIGH STRETCH

BENEFITS Besides being a tension releaser, this exercise removes stiffness and firms and tones the thighs and legs.

THE EXERCISE Sit on the floor, bend your knees, and press the soles of your feet together.

Clasp your hands around your feet and, while pulling upward on them, press your knees and thighs down as far as possible. Keep sitting up straight, close your eyes, and breathe deeply. Hold for a count of 20.

DOS AND DON'TS Don't strain or rush, and remember to breathe deeply.

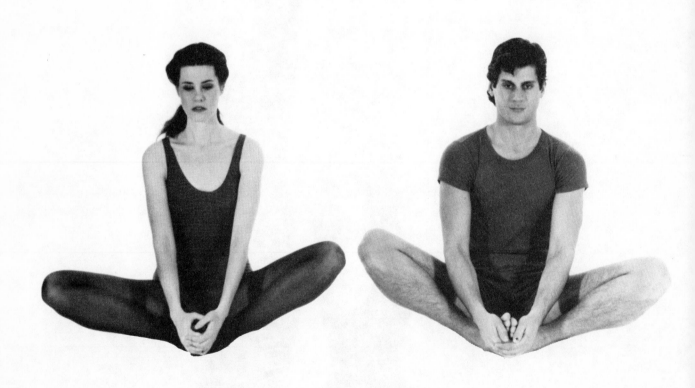

KNEE HOLD

BENEFITS This exercise releases tension as well as providing a stretch for the entire spine.

THE EXERCISE Lie flat on your backs and bring your knees into your chests.

Grasp your knees and pull them deeper into your chests, holding that position for a count of 6.

Then raise your heads and shoulders and bring your foreheads toward your knees, rolling yourselves up into a ball. Tighten all your muscles and hold for a count of 10. Then relax into your starting position.

Do this exercise 3 times.

DOS AND DON'TS Breathe deeply and evenly. Don't rush the exercise.

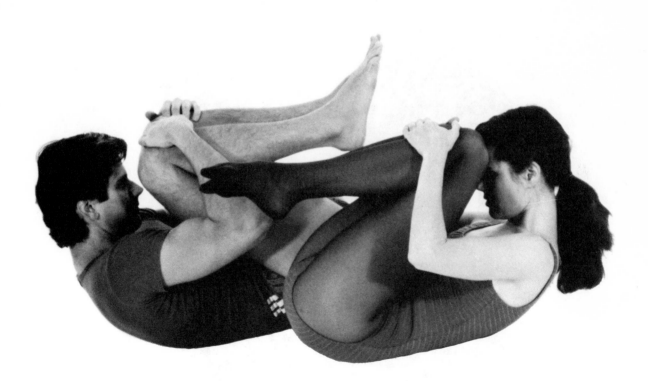

FORWARD STRETCH

BENEFITS This exercise is an excellent tension releaser and total body stretch.

THE EXERCISE Lie on your backs, arms at your sides and legs stretched out straight.

Stretch your arms behind your heads, then lift your arms, heads, and shoulders all together and fold forward toward your legs. Clasp your calves or ankles, whichever is easier, and gently pull your bodies down to your legs.

Hold for a count of 6, then roll back to your starting position.

Do this exercise 3 times.

DOS AND DON'TS Do this exercise in an easy, relaxed manner; be careful not to strain. Breathe normally.

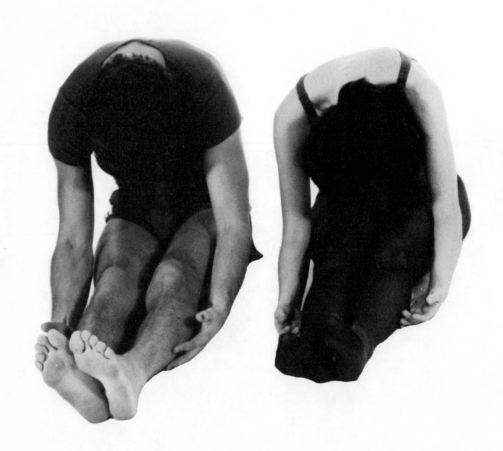

KNEE-IN

BENEFITS This exercise releases tension as well as stretching the muscles in the hip, thigh, and calf.

THE EXERCISE Lie flat on your backs, arms at your sides.

Bring one knee in toward your chest, then reach up with both arms and pull it in closer. Release the leg and straighten it up toward the ceiling. Keeping it straight, lower it to the floor. Repeat with the other leg.

Do this exercise 6 times.

DOS AND DON'TS Be sure not to rush; do this exercise in a slow and even movement. This exercise can be done with equal benefit, with either a flexed or pointed foot, with arms at the sides or in a T position.

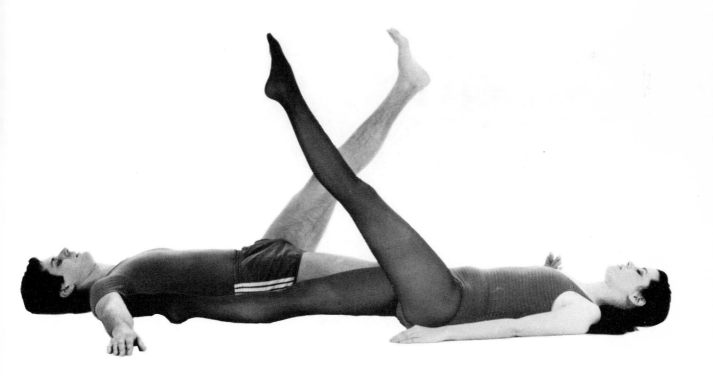

FULL BODY STRETCH

BENEFITS Besides releasing tension, this provides an excellent stretch.

THE EXERCISE Lie on your backs, legs forward and arms straight behind your heads.

Stretch your arms and legs as far as you can. Point your toes and hold for a count of 3. Then flex your feet and hands and hold for a count of 3.

Point and flex 10 times each.

DOS AND DON'TS Be sure to stretch your entire body while doing the exercise in a slow, even, and relaxed manner.

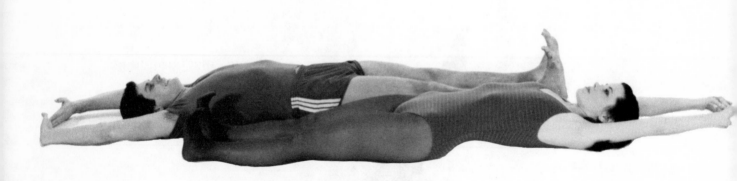

ALTERNATE SIDE STRETCH

BENEFITS Besides releasing tension, this exercise provides a terrific stretch for the chest and arms, and also aids alignment.

THE EXERCISE Lie on your backs, knees bent and arms at your sides.

First stretch your right arms straight behind you and hold for a count of 3, then return it to your side and stretch your left arms and hold for a count of 3.

Do 10 stretches right and 10 left.

DOS AND DON'TS Breathe deeply in a relaxed manner and be sure not to rush.

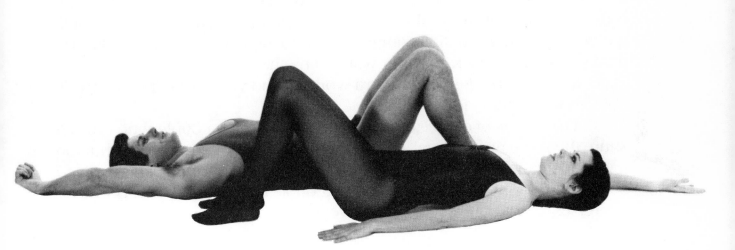

exercising alone

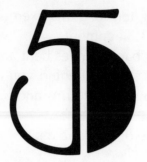

N O MATTER how well you have arranged your exercise schedule, there will inevitably be times when one partner will have to exercise alone. All sorts of things can disrupt your regular routine: a business trip, a medical emergency, separate vacations, family obligations. In such a situation, simply switch to the exercises in this chapter until you can get back together with each other.

If one of you desires an extra workout and your partner is not available, this chapter is for you, too.

This series of exercises is also intended for the couple who doesn't share the same fitness level. It provides the partner who is out of condition a way to shape up quickly and efficiently. Your fitness level can be raised sufficiently for you to embark on the couples' program if you do these exercises a half hour daily for two weeks.

THE WARM-UP

These exercises should be done one right after the other, without stopping. Be careful not to rush through the sequence, but to do each exercise smoothly and rhythmically. And remember, breathe deeply!

1. Begin in a standing position. Reach upward and out to your left with your right arm. As you do this, bend your left arm behind your back. Stretch to your left from your waist. Hold for a count of 3, then release.

Switch arm positions and repeat.

Do this exercise 3 times on each side.

2. Stand straight, reach up toward the ceiling with both arms, and bend backwards.

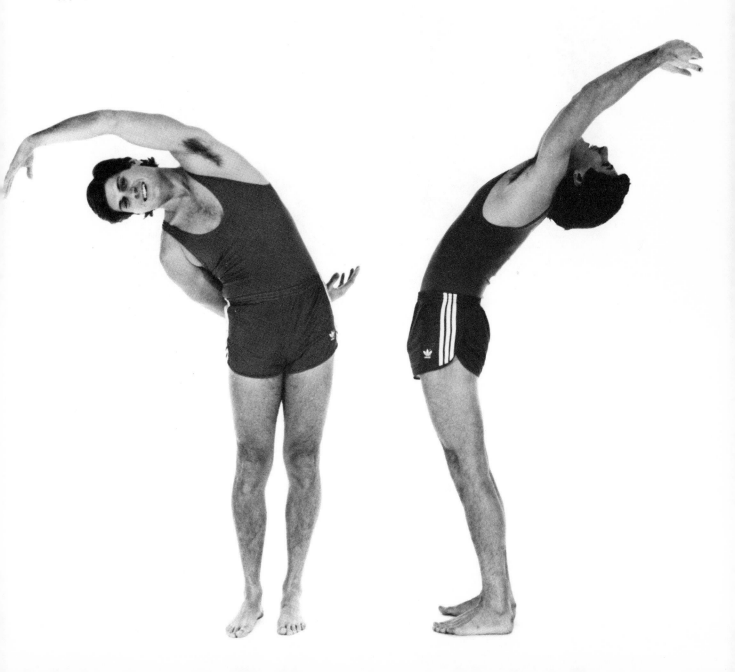

3. Then roll your body forward until your hands reach the floor.

4. With your hands touching the floor, walk your fingers forward until your body forms a pyramid. Keeping your palms on the floor, go up on your toes and down again 10 times. Finally, walk your hands back toward your legs and roll back up to a standing position.

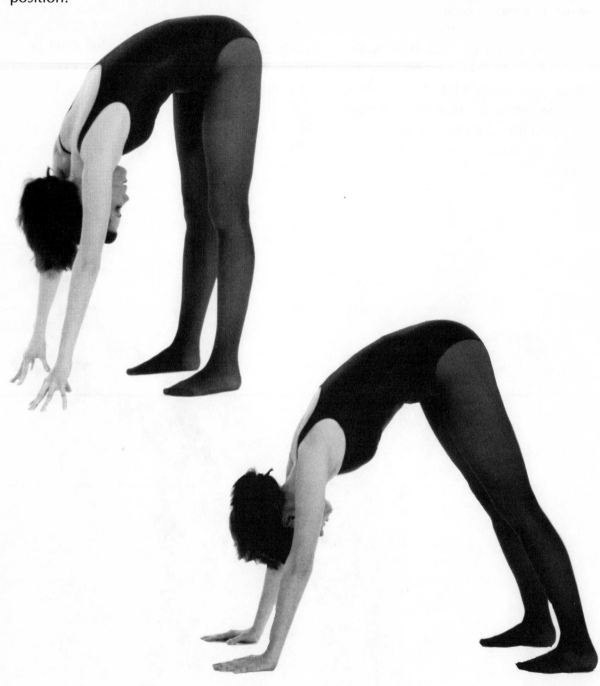

5. Bend your body forward to a flat-back position and swing your arms forward.

6. Then swing your arms back. Swing your arms forward and back in this flat-back position 10 times.

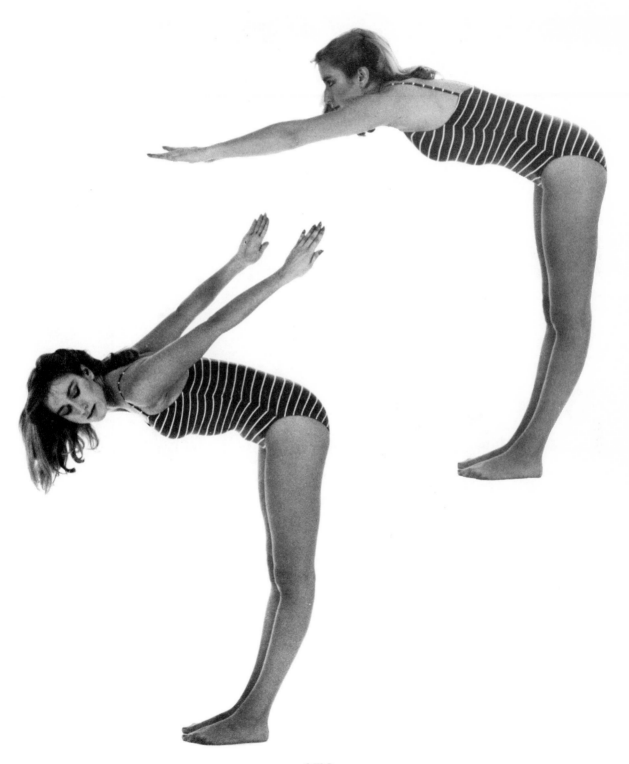

7. Then stretch your arms forward and touch the floor.

8. With your hands touching the floor, take deep breaths and bring your head in closer to your legs.

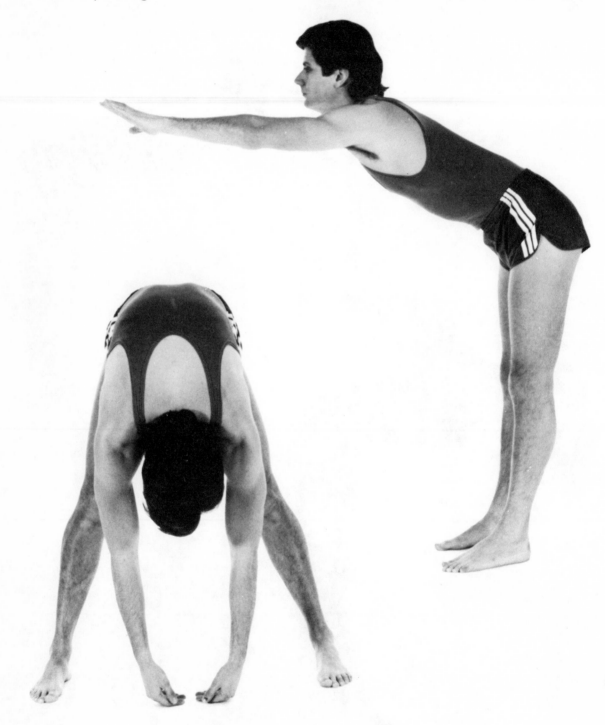

9. Now reach back and grasp your legs behind the knees, as shown. Take a deep breath and, as you exhale, hold for a count of 10.

10. Next, move your hands down along your legs to your ankles, as shown. Take a deep breath and, as you exhale, hold for a count of 10.

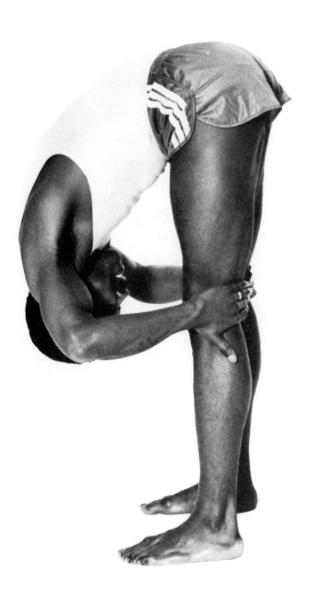 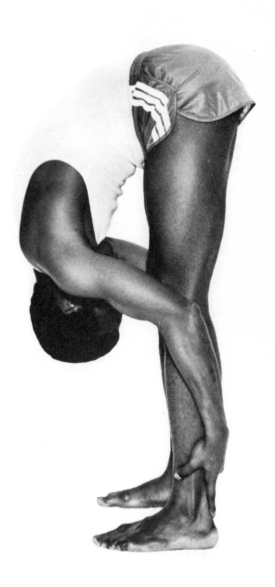

11. Roll smoothly back up and bring your arms well behind your back. Clasp your hands, arch your back so your chest is out and your head back, and pull your arms down and back.

12. Keeping your hands clasped, roll forward and swing your arms up straight behind you. Take a deep breath and, as you exhale, hold your position for a count of 10.

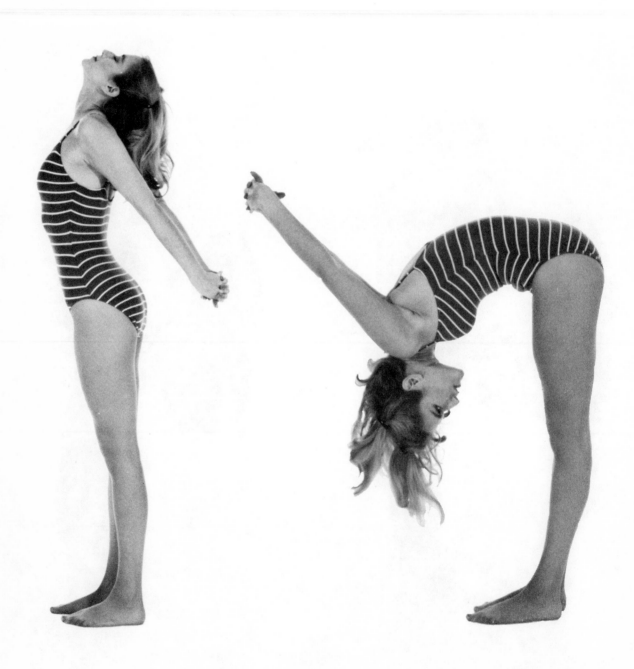

13. Unclasp your hands and bring them down to your hips. Roll back up to a flat-back position.

14. Keeping your hands on your hips, roll your body over to your right side, then to the back, then to your left side, then again to a flat-back position. Do this exercise 6 times.

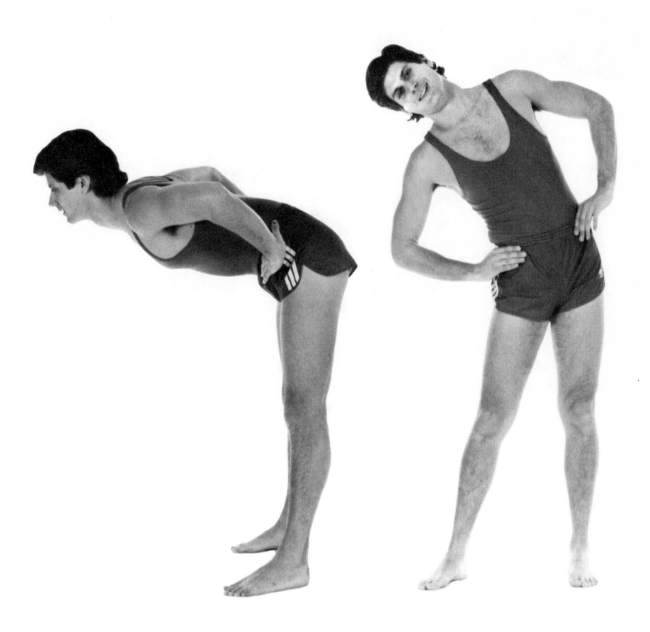

THE EXERCISES

1. Lie on your stomach with your arms at your sides, your forehead on the floor.
First lift your forehead, then your shoulders and chest. Raise your arms out to the side, keeping your fingers pointed as shown. Hold for a count of 10, then lower yourself to your original position.

Do this exercise 3 times.

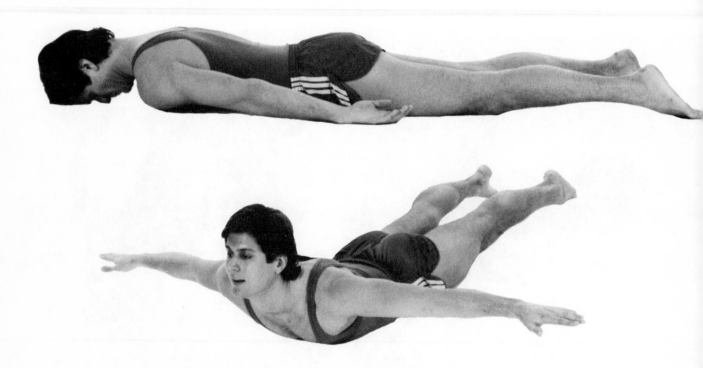

2. Lift your head, then your shoulders and chest again. Raise your arms, with your hands pointing back toward your feet, then swing them out to the side and hold for a count of 10. Swing them to the front and hold for a count of 10. Return your arms to your sides, then lower and relax.

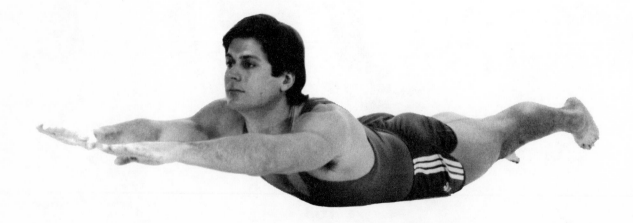

3. Lie on your stomach, your arms bent, palms next to your shoulders. Bend your knees and point your feet upward.

Push up with your hands to lift up your chest, as shown, then lower yourself back to the floor.

Do this exercise 10 times at first. Gradually build up to 30 times.

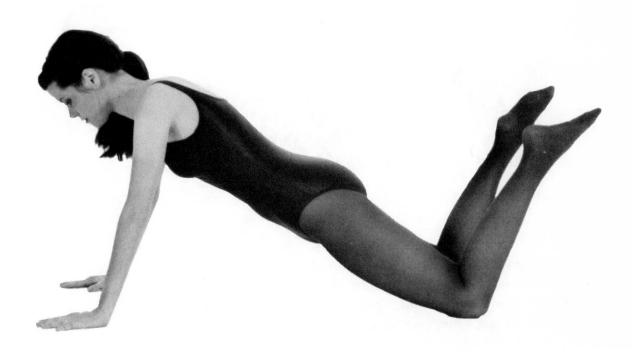

4. Lie on your back, your knees bent, your feet pressed to the floor. Place your hands on the back of your head with your elbows out to the sides.

Pull your elbows forward and, pressing your lower back to the floor and keeping your abdomen tight, lift your head and shoulders. Hold for a count of 10, then roll gently back to the floor.

Do this exercise 3 times.

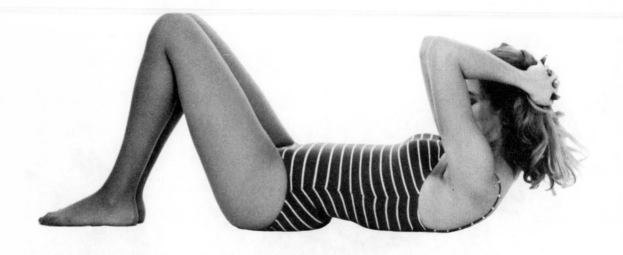

5. Lie on your back, pull your knees into your chest, and grasp them. As you do so, lift up your head and shoulders and bring your forehead to your knees. Tighten all your muscles and hold for a count of 10.

Reach your arms forward, keeping them parallel to the floor. Keeping one knee pressed against your forehead, push the other leg out and forward, keeping it parallel to and about six inches above the floor. Reverse knees and repeat.

Do this exercise 30 times, resting between each set of 10 for the count of 10.

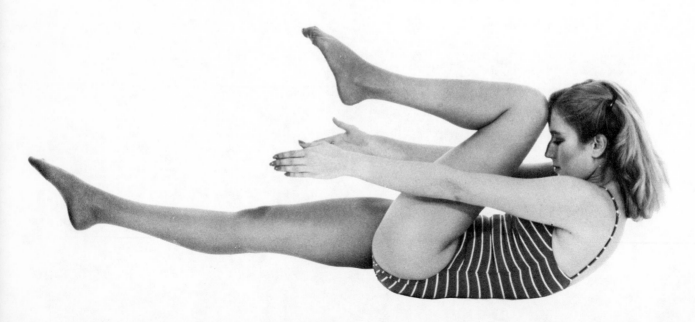

6. Sit with your knees bent, your feet pressed firmly to the floor, and your arms outstretched parallel to the floor.

Bring your chin into your chest and roll back slowly, stopping at the small of your back. Return to your original sitting position.

Do this exercise 8 times.

7. In the same sitting position, roll all the way down on the floor and stretch your arms out behind your head. Then press your lower back to the floor and raise your arms and shoulders. Come up as far as you can.

Do this exercise 8 times.

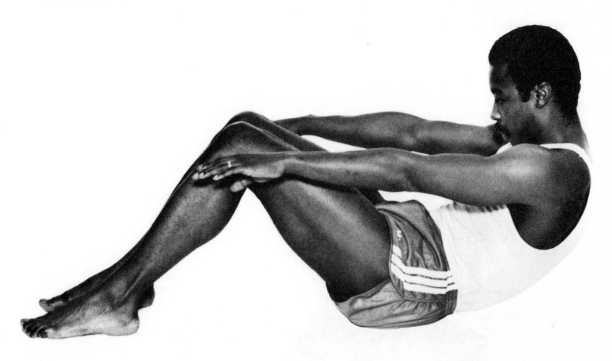

8. Sit on the floor with your legs stretched open to the sides and your toes pointed.

Keeping your back straight and your abdomen tight, stretch your arms straight up. Then bend forward and, spreading your arms apart, touch your left toe with your left hand, your right toe with your right hand. Keep leaning forward and bring your arms together. Stretch them forward in front of you with the palms flat against each other. Then sweep your arms up over your head and straighten your back.

Do this exercise 10 times at a rapid pace.

9. Sit with your legs stretched open to the sides.

Bend your body to the right and, as you do so, stretch your arms straight out over your head and parallel to the floor, as shown. Next, roll your body toward your right

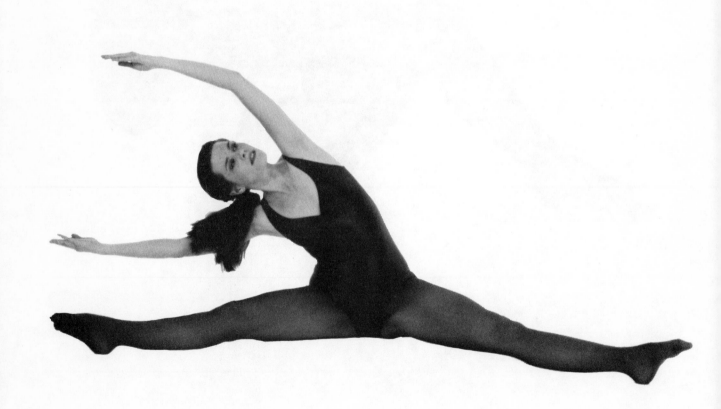

knee and touch your ankle with both hands. Then roll to the center, with your arms on the floor, as shown. For even greater flexibility, flex your feet and exhale into the

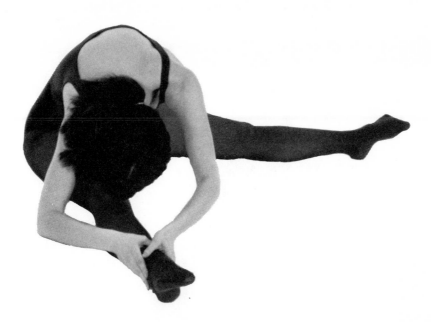

stretch. Then roll over to your left knee, touching your ankle with both hands. Finally, stretch your arms out to the sides and lift up and back to your original position. The entire sequence should be done as one flowing motion.

Do this exercise 10 times, alternating the side you start with.

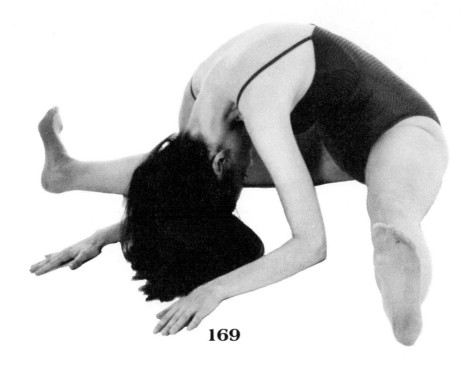

10. Lie on your left side, your head resting on your left hand and your right hand on the floor in front of your chest. Raise your right leg as far as possible and then lower it to about twelve inches above the floor. Do this exercise rapidly 10 times.

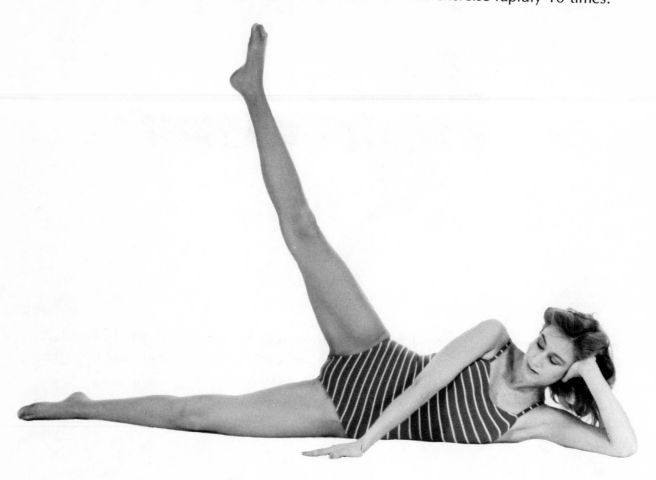

11. Still lying on your left side with both legs together, bend your right knee and pull it into your chest. Then push your leg straight back to its original position. Do this 10 times.

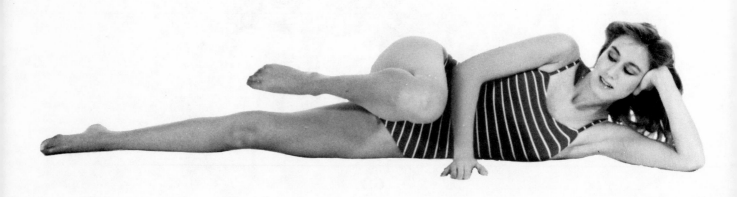

12. With your right leg raised about a foot above your left leg, swing it as far backward, then as far forward as you can (keeping it and your back straight). Do this exercise rapidly, but with control, 10 times.

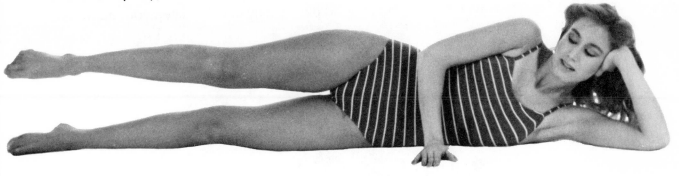

13. End the last swing with your leg in a forward position, then point your toe down and your heel up, as shown. Move your leg up and down 10 times.

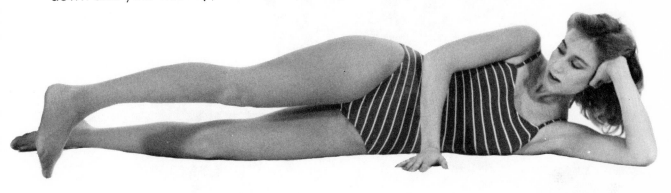

14. Bend your right knee and place that foot on the floor in front of your left knee. Then lift your left leg 10 times, as shown.

Roll over onto your right side and repeat the entire sequence.

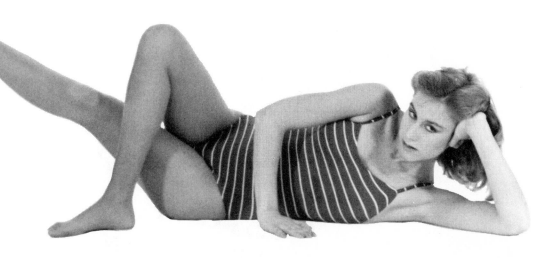

15. Kneel with your hands on the floor in front of you, as shown. Maintain a flat-back position throughout; do not arch or sway your back.

Pull your left knee up into your forehead and then stretch the leg straight out and up behind you. As you do so, lift your head as high as you can and keep your abdomen tight.

Switch legs and repeat.

Do this exercise 10 times.

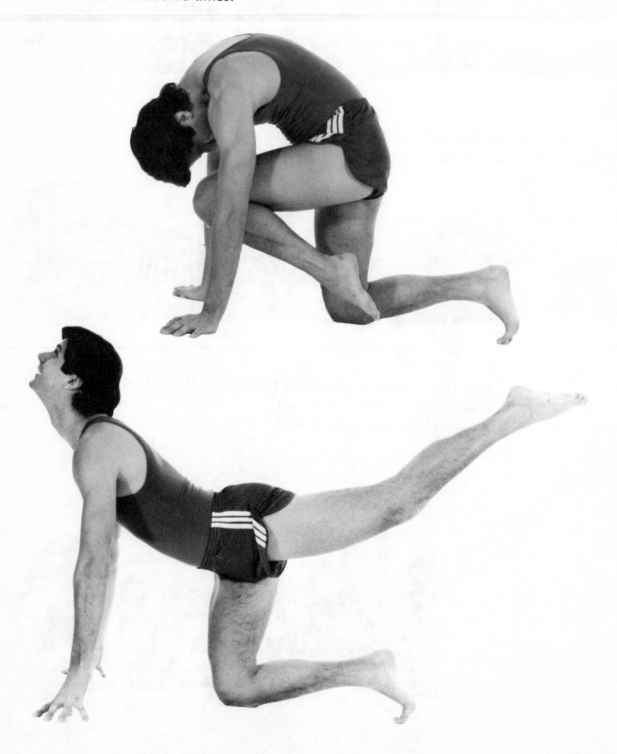

16. Lie flat on your back with your hands at the back of your head. Lift up your head and shoulders, pulling your elbows toward the center. Pull your left knee in toward your elbows while you stretch the right leg forward (making sure to keep it off the ground).

Return to the floor, switch legs, and repeat.

Do this exercise 10 times for each leg.

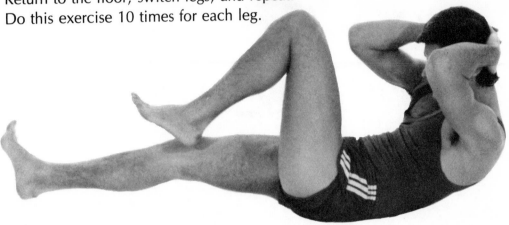

17. Lie on your back with your arms in a T.

Pull your knees into your chest, then roll your knees over to the right side, then to the left side. If you can, touch the ground with your knees when you roll over. But you *must* keep your shoulders and arms pressed to the floor.

Do this exercise 6 times.

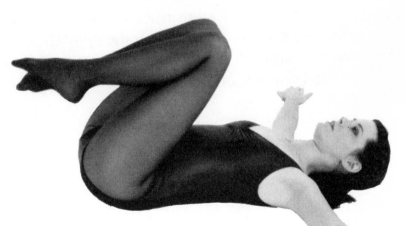

COOL-DOWN

After completing this entire series, turn to the cool-down portion of the regular couples' program on page 144. Follow the cool–down segment as directed.

special cases: exercises for sports and problem spots

6

T HE STRETCHING EXERCISES in this chapter were developed to help you with any sports program you are engaged in as well as with any physical problem spots you may have. They are a pleasant addition to your exercise program. There is no limit to the number of times these exercises may be performed daily. Do them before you undertake any vigorous exercise or whenever the spirit moves you. These exercises will provide a smooth, easy transition to any form of strenuous physical activity. Suggestions are made for which sports each exercise is most beneficial.

These exercises will also help to alleviate painful backaches and the discomfort in arthritic hands, stiff joints, and other problem areas. They can also help if you are feeling generally stiff and achey as the result of too much standing or sitting or an accumulation of nervous tension and muscular tightness. Poor posture, overweight, and a long-term neglect of the body's basic exercise needs also contribute to aches and stiffness and they can lead to a serious lack of abdominal strength—often the real culprit where lower back pain is concerned. (All of this, naturally, is based on the assumption that you have had a complete physical and that your doctor has given you a clean bill of health.)

If back pain is the problem, additional work with chapter 5, "Exercising Alone," would be an excellent way to build up abdominal strength, and exercises for the hips, buttocks, and midriff will also be useful. During your daily routine, you can exercise without anyone's notice by constantly contracting the abdominal muscles. This will not only flatten the stomach but will improve posture as well. As you go through the day, always try to keep your head in line with your spine, whether you're standing, sitting, or lying down. Walk and stand tall, with your stomach tight and your chest and rib cage lifted up and away from your hips.

As you go through the exercises in this chapter, remember to take it slow and easy! Avoid sudden jerky movements and be especially careful not to twist your body quickly from side to side. *Think* before you move! A gentle rhythm is helpful, but pronounced bouncing is not; you should feel peaceful and relaxed doing these exercises. This is not the time to compete with yourself or with each other. Your purpose here is to release muscular tension and allow your body freer movement, whether you're preparing to ski down a mountain or just to get through the day. Concentrate on the areas of your body that are the most troublesome for you. Don't force your body into an extreme stretch; simply do each exercise in the way that feels most comfortable to you. Stretching should not be painful; if you try to do too much too soon you will only injure yourself. Listen to your body. It will tell you quite clearly when it's ready for the next plateau.

And of course, remember to breathe deeply and naturally, exhaling into each stretch.

Happy exercising!

NECK, SHOULDERS, AND CHEST

Do the following exercises if you have any problems with your neck, shoulders, or chest and before participation in any sport that involves quick twisting, lifting, or stretching of your head, neck, shoulders, arms, or chest, for example baseball, softball, tennis, and racketball.

1. Stand with legs a hip's width apart. Bend over and swing your arms back as far as they will go. Keep your arms straight and press your palms toward each other 10 times.

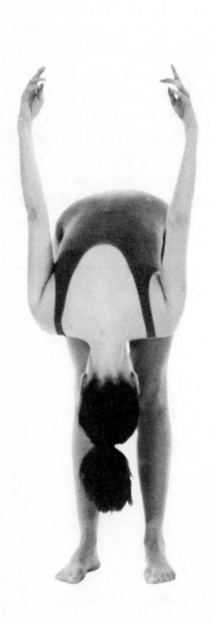
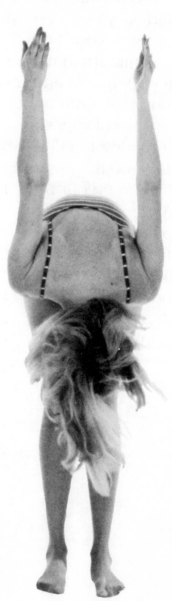

2. Sit on the floor, your legs crossed tailor-fashion. Grasp your left wrist and bend over to the right side, keeping your arms up and slightly back. Pull gently on the grasped wrist 10 times. Reverse and repeat with your left side.

3. Sit on the floor, your legs crossed tailor-fashion. Bend your body forward, touching your head to the floor. As you do so, clasp your hands behind your back and, keeping your arms straight, lift them as high as you can without lifting your buttocks from the floor. Hold the position for a count of 10.

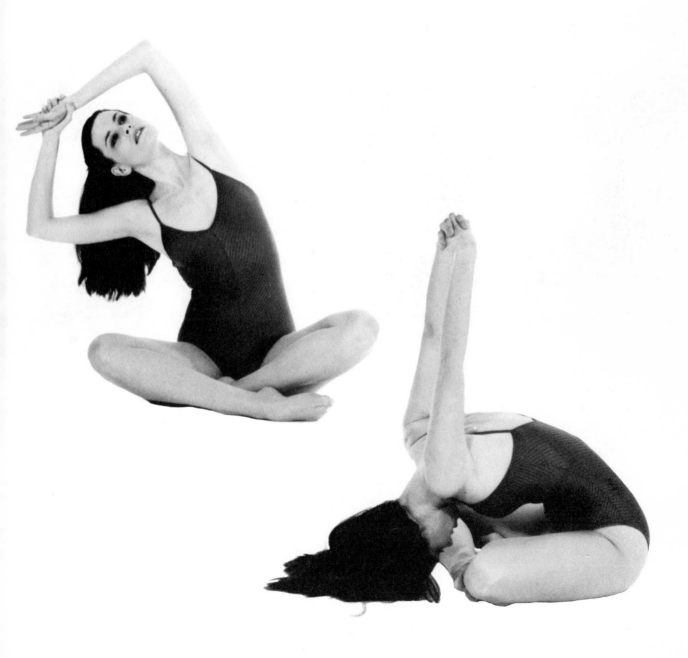

4. Lie on your back and pull your knees in toward your chest. Cross your arms over your chest and press your hands to the floor next to your ears, as shown. Hold for a count of 10.

5. Stand with your arms extended overhead, crossed at the wrist and with your palms together. Stretch your arms upward and slightly back. Hold for a count of 10, then bring your hands down. Do this exercise 3 times.

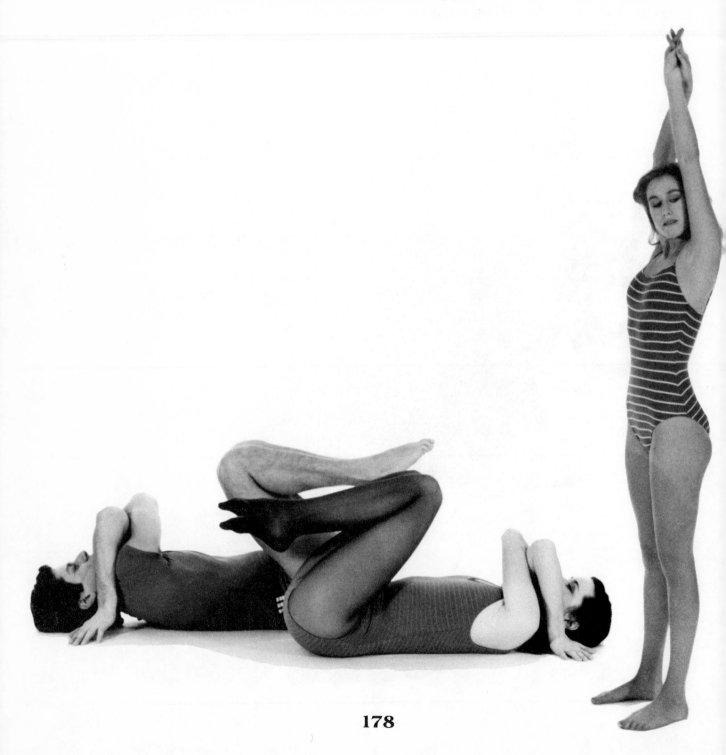

6. Standing, bring your arms overhead, and grasp your right elbow with your left hand. Gently and slowly pull the elbow behind your head as you stretch to the left. Hold the position for a count of 15, then repeat with the left elbow, stretching right.

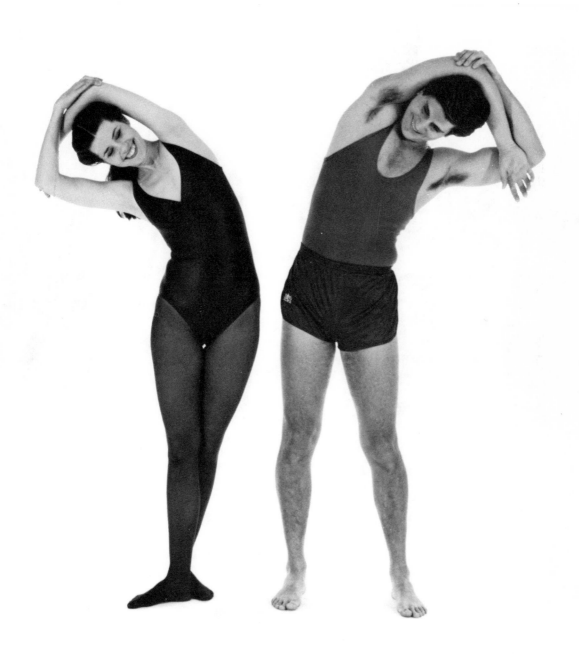

7. Standing, bring your arms behind your back and interlace your fingers. Slowly turn your elbows inward so they face each other as you straighten your arms, as shown. Next, keeping them straight, lift your arms up behind you until you feel a stretch in your arms and shoulders. Hold this position for a count of 20.

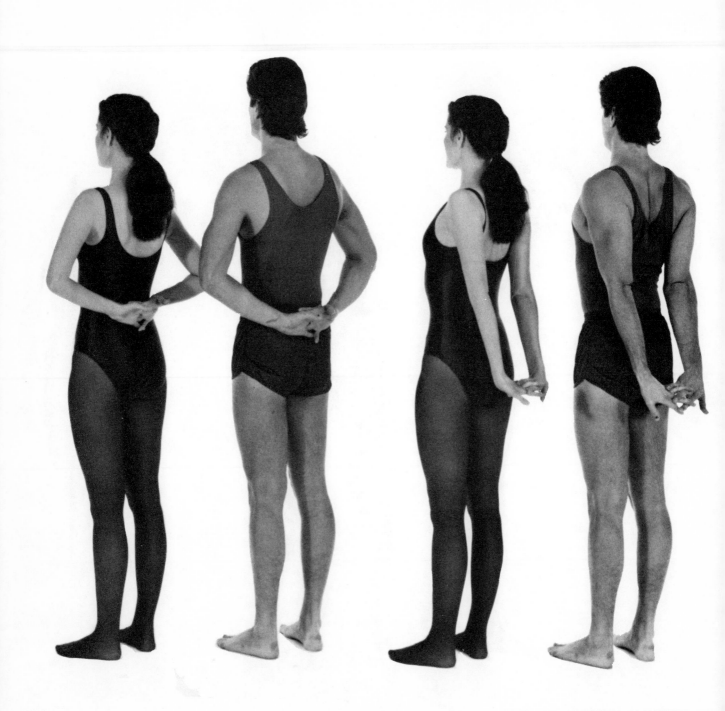

8. Standing, bring your right hand over your head and place it on the left cheek. Gently pull 10 times. Repeat with your left hand on your right cheek.

9. Stand facing forward. Turn your head and bring your chin over your left shoulder, keeping it at right angles to that shoulder. Then drop your chin toward the shoulder. Raise and drop your chin 10 times, then resume your original forward-facing position and repeat with your right shoulder.

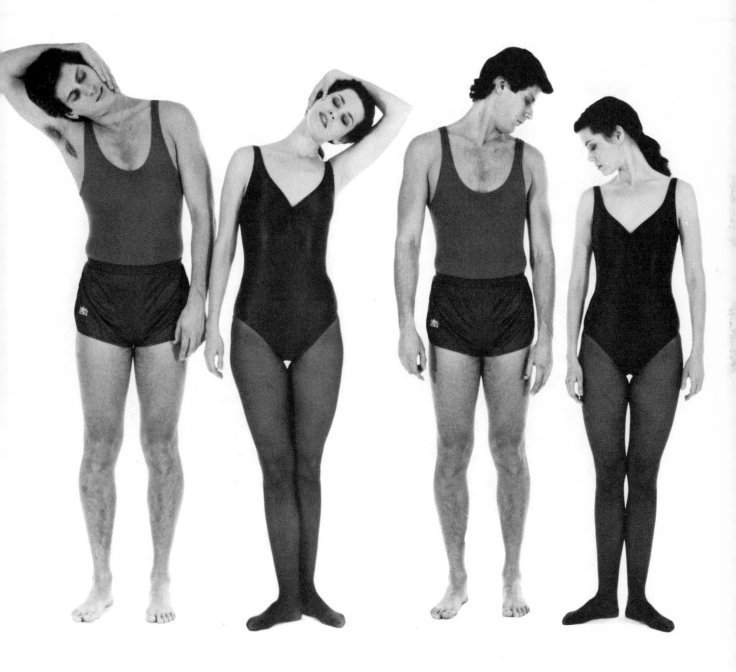

LOWER BACK, ABDOMEN, AND HIPS

These exercises are especially beneficial for problems with your lower back, abdomen, and hips. They are also recommended as warm-up exercises for sports that demand quick twisting movements of the hips, lower back, and pelvis, such as basketball, golf, cycling, football, or gymnastics. You can become a candidate for lower back injuries if you don't keep these areas supple. If the muscles in the lower back and hips are called upon to exert energy before they are properly warmed up, they could tear or strain.

1. Sit on the floor, bend your knees, and bring the soles of your feet together, holding them with your hands. Then gently push your knees down and release, as shown, 10 times. Don't force it.

This exercise provides an easy stretch through your inner thighs, abdomen, and groin, and helps to eliminate tension in your lower back.

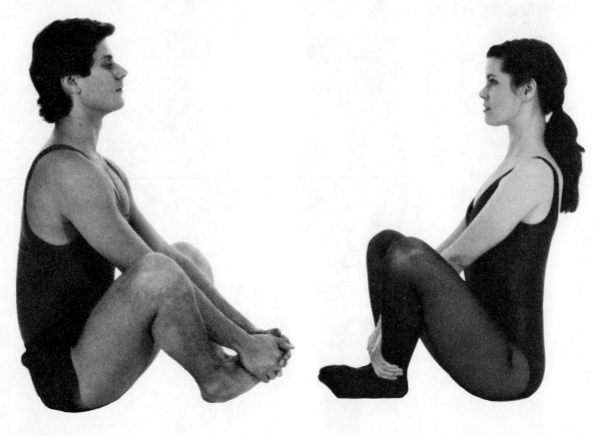

2. Lie on your back with your knees bent and your arms flat at your sides. Press your lower back to the floor, keeping your abdomen tight, and hold for a count of 10. Then arch your lower back, as shown, and hold for a count of 10. Release the arch and ease down; do not lift your head.

This exercise releases tension throughout your lower back.

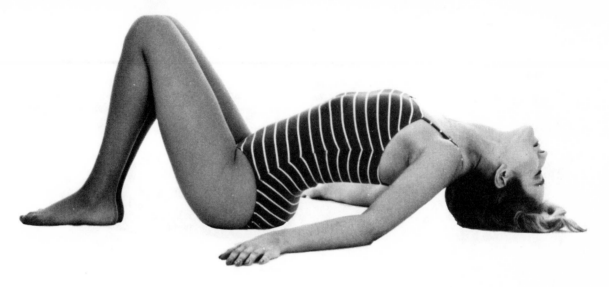

3. Lie flat on your back, your legs straight and your arms stretched back behind your head. Keeping your shoulders pressed to the floor, lift your right arm and right leg vertically into the air. Hold for a count of 10. Lower, then lift your left arm and left leg.

This exercise stretches your entire body, but especially your hips and legs.

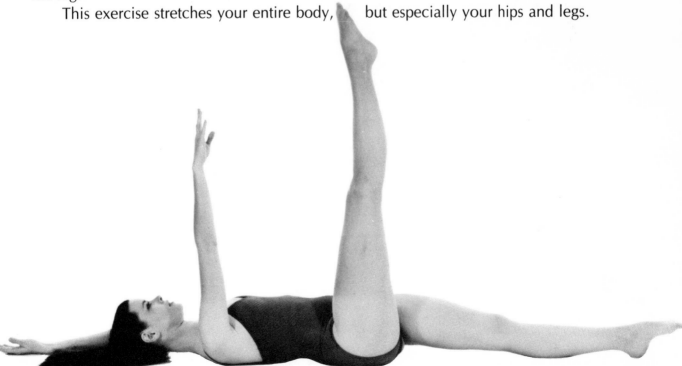

4. Lie on your back with your knees bent and your feet pressed to the floor. Interlace your fingers on the back of your head and slowly pull your head forward with your arms until you can feel a stretch at the back of your head and neck. Hold this position for a count of 10. Do this exercise 3 times.

This exercise strengthens your abdomen and releases tension in your upper back.

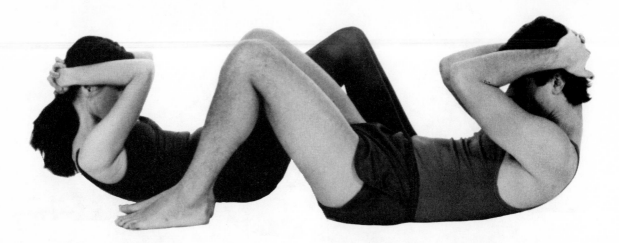

5. Lie on your back, your arms spread out to the sides, your knees bent. Lift your left leg over your right. Then, keeping your upper back, head, and shoulders flat on the floor, use the left leg to push the right one down toward the floor, as shown, until you can feel a stretch in your hips and lower back. Hold this position for a count of 30. Then repeat this exercise on the other side.

This exercise releases tension in your lower back.

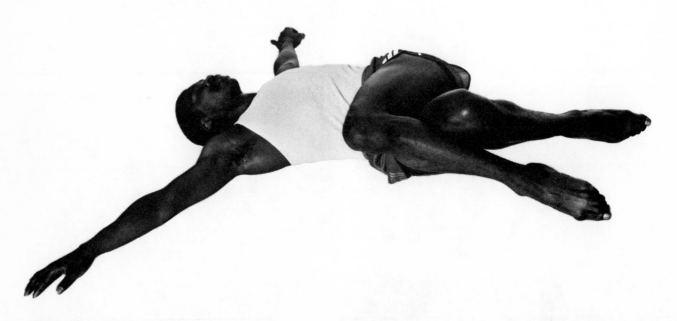

LEGS, ANKLES, AND FEET

Try these exercises if you have any problems with your legs, ankles, or feet, as well as to prepare yourself for participating in such sports as running or jogging, cross-country or downhill skiing, soccer, surfing, swimming, ice hockey, or ice or roller skating. All of these sports demand that your thighs, knees, and feet be strong and flexible. If there's a lack of flexibility, injuries such as torn ligaments, ripped cartilage, pinched nerves, or pulled hamstrings could occur. Or you might fall and cause other injuries, ranging all the way from bruised knees to broken bones.

1. From a standing position, squat down, keeping your feet flat on the ground (if possible) and your toes pointed out. Your knees should be tucked just outside your shoulders and positioned directly above your big toes. Hold this position for a count of 30.

This is a very good exercise for stretching the front of your lower legs, your knees, ankles, and Achilles tendons, and back.

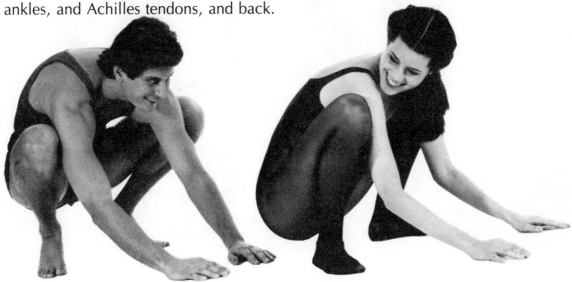

2. Lie on your stomach. Reach behind you with your left hand to grasp the top of your right foot. Gently pull your right heel toward the middle of your buttocks. Hold this position for a count of 10. Repeat with your right arm and left foot.

This exercise stretches your legs, chest, and shoulders.

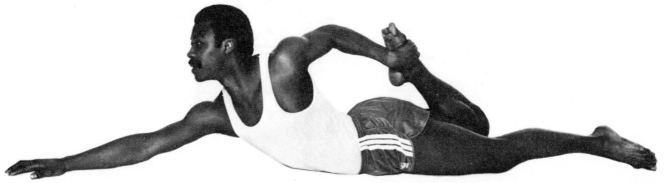

3. Sit on the floor with your knees bent and the soles of your feet together and gently relax yourself forward, placing your palms on the floor in front of your feet, as shown. Leading with your hips, relax and lower your torso toward the floor. Hold this position for a count of 10. Do this exercise 3 times.

This exercise is particularly effective in stretching your inner thighs and relaxing your lower back.

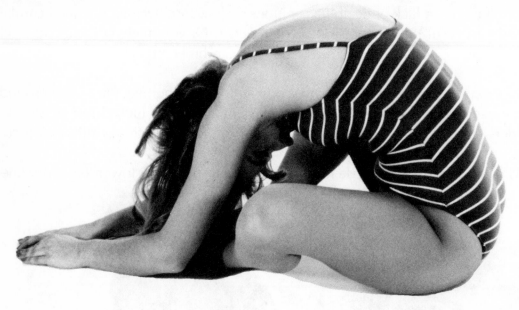

4. Sit on the floor and stretch your legs open to the side, keeping your feet flexed. Put your hands on the back of your head and pull forward. Lower your torso forward, leading with your hips. Hold the position for a count of 10, then return to your sitting up position. Do this exercise 3 times.

This exercise stretches your inner thighs, hips, and entire spine.

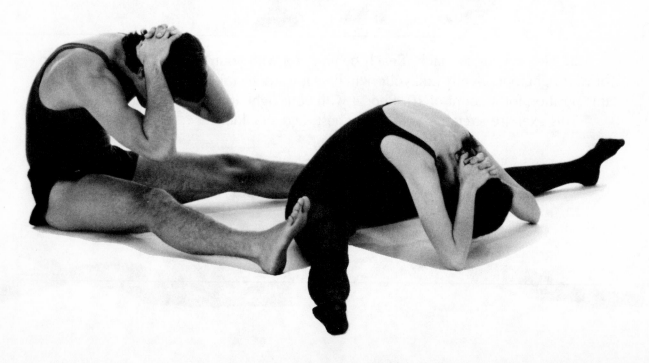

5. Kneel down and move your left leg forward until the knee is over or a few inches in front of your ankle. Stretch your right leg straight back behind you, as shown, with only your toes touching the floor. Now lower the front of your left hip downward to create an easy stretch. Hold this position for a count of 30. Repeat with your right leg forward and your left leg back.

This exercise is an excellent stretch for your thighs and hips, and promotes flexibility through the legs and hips.

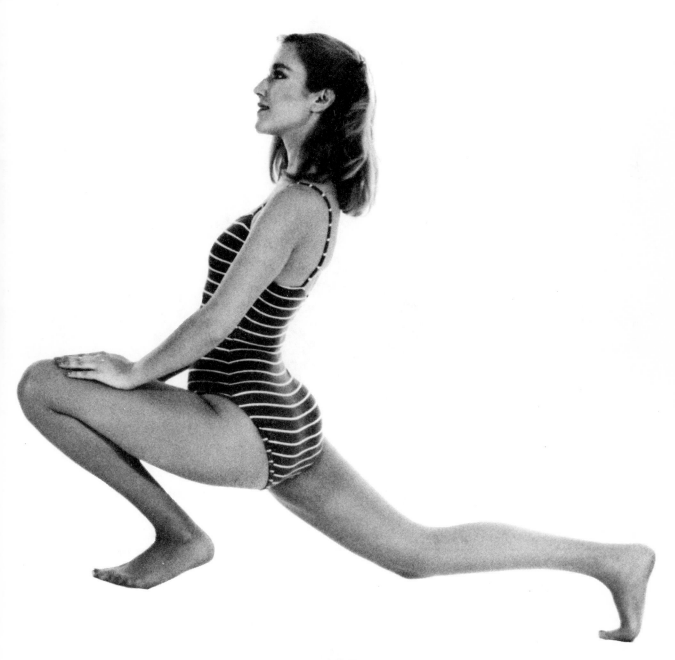

6. Lie flat on your back. Supporting your back with your hands, bring your body up into a shoulder stand, as shown. Maintaining control at all times, lower your left leg and lift it again, then lower and lift your right leg. Do this exercise 6 times. Roll back down slowly, knees to chest, to avoid jerking your body.

This is a terrific stretch for your legs and hips.

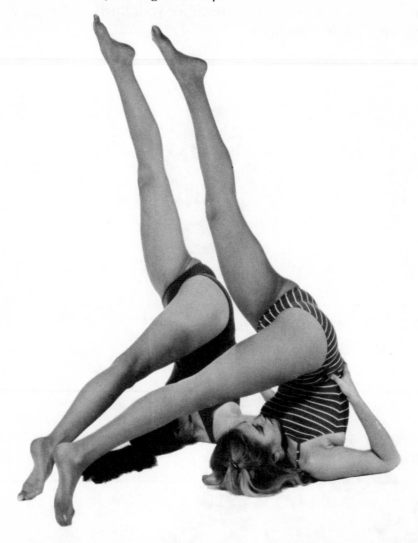

7. Lie on your back, hands clasped above your head, the soles of your feet pressed together and your knees bent out to the sides. Gently press the knees toward the floor in a rocking motion 10 times.

This is a good stretch for your inner thighs and hips, and relaxes your entire body as well.

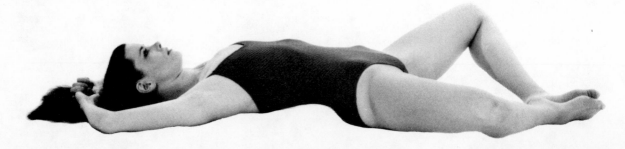

unwinding together

7

BEFORE TAKING his first class, one of my students insisted, "I'm here to firm my body! I've no time for this relaxation garbage!" This was said while he twisted his hands, tapped his foot, and kept glancing nervously from side to side. So at first I created a program for him that concentrated only on exercise . . . even though his concentration was non-existent! Not surprisingly, his progress was slow, very slow. Gradually I introduced the "relaxation garbage" into his program and watched with interest. His concentration improved, and he began to get more and more out of the exercise sessions. Not long after that he sheepishly admitted that his chronic sleep problems had eased and there was a definite improvement in his performance at work—both in quantity and quality! Not to mention that somehow things with his girl friend had gotten better, much, much better. "Best of all," he reported, "I feel ten years younger!"

There are many misconceptions about just what relaxation is. So often I hear people fearfully say, "Don't teach me how to relax! I have more work to do *now* than I can handle. If I slow down it will never get done!" But to be relaxed does not mean to be lazy. The simple fact is that once you know *how* to focus, *how* to center, *how* to function in an orderly and organized fashion, you will accomplish *more* each day, not less! It may sound strange, but it's true: Relax, you'll get more done!

There is so much stress in today's world that most of us have forgotten how to relax! Yet not all stress is bad. We all experience emotions that are exhilarating: winning at tennis, watching an exciting movie, making love—all of these involve stress and tension, but it's the healthy kind. The kind that can energize you, give you a rosy, healthy, happy glow, and often even relax you! It's the other kind of stress you have to watch out for, the kind that produces intense or persistent anger and annoyance, fear, frustration, or worry. We're surrounded by all kinds of bad-stress-producing situations: air and noise pollution, demanding jobs, family problems, financial difficulties, rising crime rates, explosive international crises, and on and on. It never stops!

When you suffer from this kind of stress, it's hardly surprising that it adversely affects your body as well as your mind. My student who didn't have time for "this relaxation garbage" was so tense that he was at first totally unable to let go and stretch. It was obvious to me that the only way he could handle all his stress was to keep a "tight grip" on himself. His body remained rigid, no matter how hard he tried to relax. Ironically, his need to keep it all together was so overwhelming that he could hardly move!

His problem is far from uncommon. Many of us rebel against the very idea of relaxation when we are tense or overwrought. Subconsciously we feel that everything will fall apart if we dare to let go. Yet unless we can teach ourselves to let go of this stress, the effect on our minds and bodies can be devastating. We wind up suffering from one or more of these stress-induced symptoms: irritability, depression, sleeplessness, appetite loss or, conversely, binge eating, heart palpitations, headaches, indigestion. Many stress-afflicted people are plagued with ailments ranging from simple nervous twitching to peptic ulcers, high blood pressure, hives, spastic colon, nausea, and vomiting. Sadly, some people react to stress by building emotional walls around themselves, cutting themselves off from their friends and loved ones even though they don't really intend to—and exactly when they need them most! Still others are so desperate that they resort to alcohol or drugs to make it through the day.

What can you do to manage stress? Actually, quite a lot. First, you can accept the fact that there are some sources of stress that won't go away no matter what you do. You can scowl and mumble under your breath as you are jostled while walking down a crowded street, or try to shut out the noise of angry drivers blowing horns or the wail of ambulance or fire engine or police car sirens. You can pretend you're not afraid as you walk down into the subway or carry the garbage down the dark driveway late at night. But no matter what you do, you can't make these things go away. Your basic rule should be: *Don't waste energy on wishing you could change things that are totally out of your control.*

To win the battle against stress, you must focus on areas that you *can* change and control, areas in yourself: your body, your self-image, your relationships with your friends, family, loved ones. Everyone knows that personal relationships are more important than ever in these stressful times. And yet, as one of my students said, "It's impossible for me to get close when I'm always feeling so worried and nervous!" Impossible, yet this closeness is what we seem to need and desire the most.

But don't despair, there's good news! You don't have to feel worried and nervous and cut off from the very people who should be closest to you. Even as you work through the fitness program in this book, you will find yourself easing up, letting down those useless emotional defenses, becoming closer to and more intimate with your partner and the other people in your life. To maximize this result, and to help you get the most out of the couples' fitness program, we have provided the special relaxation exercises in this chapter. Once you master these—and remember, *mastering* in this context really means learning how to let go—you will be well on the way to a serene, productive, and healthy life-style.

Before you start, however, take some time to observe your behavior and find out just how tense you really are. Make a few spot checks throughout the day: Are your fists clenched, jaws locked, teeth grinding? Observe your hands: Do you bite your nails? Tap your fingers? As you make these observations, consciously relax your fists, your jaws, whatever part of your body is tense. A little while later, check yourself again. Then consciously relax again. This is a simple first step. Go one step farther and observe your partner or co-worker. Don't be surprised if he or she shows visible signs of tension too! We all do. Once you become aware of this protective tension pattern and begin to let it go you will find that it's just as natural to relax. When you're on edge, waiting for the worst to happen, it doesn't matter whether the worst happens or not. Your poor exhausted body has already experienced the trauma and paid the price!

Now that you have some awareness of your level of stress and tension, practice the following relaxation techniques. If you find that your tension is getting in the way, continue to work with these techniques day after day until you have worked through it. It's important that you proceed to the couples' fitness program only *after* you have successfully lowered your stress level. Until then, work out with the "Exercising Alone" program in chapter 5.

Basic relaxation exercises

These exercises should be done with your mind focused only on the exercise. A few minutes of total involvement in one exercise will benefit you much more than ten exercises performed in a bored or distracted way!

Three-part elementary relaxation stretch

1. In a standing position, let go: Let your head hang down, your torso bend forward, your shoulders and arms slump toward the floor. Relax your knees but continue to support your body through the legs and hips. Tilt your torso farther over and, holding yourself as if you were a rag doll, shake your arms, head, and shoulders, and let all your tension fall away. Breathe deeply; if you exhale into the stretch you will have more flexibility.

2. In a standing position, tighten your face, arms, hands, chest, stomach, buttocks, thighs, legs, feet. Your entire body should be in a state of contraction. Hold for a count of 10, then release.

   After you release, let go again as in step 1.

3. In a standing position, repeat steps 1 and 2, then stretch. Stretch toward the ceiling, reaching both arms as high as you can; then stretch to the right, then to the left, then forward in a flat-back posture, and then straight up. Finally, reach as far back as you can, then relax forward and try to touch your toes. Now let go again, as in step 1.

   You can repeat this sequence any time of the day, as needed. Make sure you do the entire series with total involvement. Concentrate on what you are doing at the moment you are doing it—and on nothing else!

Before we go on to the next part of these basic relaxation exercises, let's take a moment to analyze what happened to you when you did the elementary stretch. Did you notice what a tremendous amount of energy it takes to hold a muscle in a state of contraction? Compare the tension your body felt when you tightened all your muscles with the release you experienced when you let go. Relaxation is the opposite of contraction; the exercise you have just performed intensifies each feeling so you really feel the effect of tension on the body and you really feel the release that occurs when you relax. When you stretch you draw tension away from the muscles that were constricted and instead send energy to all parts of your body. Remember to always stretch with the "let go" attitude!

When you are completely relaxed, only that energy necessary to maintain life is being used. The nerves and muscles are at rest, and energy is stored and conserved, available to be applied wherever it is truly needed. People who understand how to relax always accomplish more because they are more "fuel-efficient" than most other people. It's as though instead of twelve miles to the gallon, they are getting forty! If you are rushing around, racing your motor and spinning your wheels but going nowhere, you are wasting a tremendous amount of energy. When you are out of control mentally, both the body and the nervous system are affected. For complete well-being, you need exercise for the body and relaxation for the mind.

Simple total body relaxation

Lie flat on your back and make your mind and body as relaxed as possible. Center yourself: Spread your arms and legs out to the side an equal distance from the center of your torso; gently roll your head from side to side and then line it up with your torso. Close your eyes and listen to your breathing; allow it to become rhythmic. Each time you inhale, mentally concentrate on the number *one*. As you exhale, concentrate on completely relaxing throughout your face, torso, arms, and legs.

Continue to breathe deeply and rhythmically. Become limp and loose as you become increasingly relaxed. Concentrate on your fingers and toes; make them totally relaxed. Concentrate on the small muscles in your face, jaw, scalp, ears; make them totally relaxed. Totally relax everything. Stay in this position for ten to fifteen minutes, your eyes closed, concentrating on making yourself totally relaxed.

Before we go on to the third step in these Basic Relaxation Exercise techniques, let's analyze what happened in the relaxation sequence you just did. Did you notice you were getting a deep feeling of self-control and peace, both mental and physical, as you did this exercise? As this exercise should have demonstrated to you, the mind and its thoughts are deeply connected to the body and its ability to remain calm. Through the simple expedient of focusing your mind on a number or syllable and regulating your breathing, your mind automatically begins to gentle your overwrought nerves and counteract the muscle-bound condition that occurs when you are tense and anxious.

If at first your mind refuses to remain focused, don't despair. Let it jump around, but keep gently pulling it back under your control. It might take some effort at first, but gradually, with each subsequent attempt, you will find it responding to your instructions more readily. Once you have acquired this control over your inner mental processes, you will no longer be at the mercy of negative thoughts or worries, real or imagined. Eventually, you will be able to relax and focus *at will*.

Simple concentration exercise

Place an object on the floor. It should be something simple and familiar, a flower in a vase or a lighted candle, for instance. Sit on the floor with the object in front of you, your legs crossed tailor-fashion, your hands placed comfortably on your knees. Relax your body and take a few deep breaths. Concentrate your attention on the object. Consider its size, shape, and color. Try to feel its texture with your mind. Close your eyes and re-create the object in your mind's eye exactly as you saw it. Once you have this image in your mind, concentrate on it for a few seconds, then open your eyes. Repeat the exercise. Each time you close your eyes, try to re-create the object in as much detail as possible. Continue doing this for five to ten minutes.

Don't let the apparent simplicity of these three basic relaxation exercises mislead you. Just as you undertake a physical exercise program step by step, so must you proceed in mental conditioning. Before you can successfully train yourself in more complex mental exercises* you must first be able to attain total concentration and complete relaxation and a body with no tension blocks. How you react to these exercises will reveal a good deal about your present level of tension and about your ability to relax at will.

How did you do? If you found that you had good control over yourself and were able to relax rather easily, continue with the complete fitness program. If you found these exercises difficult, continue working with them until you feel totally at ease. In either case, it might be a smart idea to incorporate them as a regular prelude to your exercise program. You should make a point of practicing these techniques as often as you can. They're wonderful for releasing tension and you can do them just about anywhere.

Massage

Another wonderful relaxation technique is massage. It's also a terrific way to get closer together, both physically and emotionally! I would strongly recommend that at least once a week you and your partner schedule a massage session after your exercise session. One week you can give the massage, the next week you can receive it.

Since there are so very many different kinds of massage, here I'll just give you the basics—certainly enough to get you off to a good start! If you want to explore further, consult the suggested reading list which begins on page 208.

First and foremost, you should be relaxed. Concentrate only on what you are doing to your partner. Your partner should be relaxed and concentrating on what he or she is feeling. This is no time for talking. The skin is your most sensitive organ, so relax and enjoy the sensations! Some people like to use oil or cream for massage. It does tend to make the touch less delicate and sensitive, however, since it forms a barrier between hands and body. It's a matter of personal preference; try it both

*See the suggested reading list (pages 208–210) for books on more complex techniques.

ways and see which you enjoy most. Naturally, it's best for the person receiving the massage to be naked.

There are three basic massage techniques: stroking, rolling, and kneading.

Stroking can be soothing or stimulating, depending on the pressure you exert and the rate and length of your strokes. Place the palm of your hand gently on the skin and move it in any direction, following or even overlapping with the other hand to give the feeling of a series of hands. Both hands should slide easily over the area being massaged, closely follow its contours, and just as delicately leave it.

Rolling starts by grasping the skin as if you are picking it up. Roll your thumbs flat on the skin, exerting a gentle but firm pressure, and push a roll of the underlying fat toward the forefingers. Repeat all over the area in any direction.

Kneading is done by alternately pressing and relaxing pressure from the palms on the muscles beneath them.

Following are directions for the three basic massages most people like to have.

Foot massage

This is a highly sensual experience, which everyone seems to enjoy. First sponge the feet with warm water and soap and pat dry with a thick towel. Sit opposite your partner, who should be leaning back in a comfortable chair. Cover your lap with a towel and support one foot on it.

Place the palm of one hand on the sole of the foot. Place the other hand gently on the top of the foot and stroke both hands toward the heel. Repeat the stroking a few times, beginning the stroke with the fingertips only and then gradually hugging the foot closely with both palms.

Place the tips of the three middle fingers of each hand just in front of and below each ankle bone and knead with fingers deeply and thoroughly all around the indentation between these bones and the heel. Repeat several times, gradually making your fingertips fit deeply but comfortably into either side of the ankle joint.

Stroke the top and the sole of the foot and then stroke each toe separately with the middle fingertip of each hand, working down the toe from the side of the nail to the junction of the toe with the foot.

Place your hands so that the palms are across the sole of the foot and the two thumbs across the roots of the toes. Follow the contours of the foot carefully, kneading toward the ankle with your thumbs. Do this fairly lightly, as the top of the foot is rather bony.

Now do the other foot.

Facial massage

This massage technique helps to drain the fluid from the sinus cavities.

Place your fingertips on the center of your partner's chin and, pressing gently down, knead toward the ear. Create a little bulge of flesh at the pads of the moving fingers. Work first along the jawline; next, from the nostrils to the ear; then over the cheekbones just under the eyes. Never massage the eye socket; it's too delicate. Always massage up and out toward the ears.

Massage the forehead. First work from the bridge of the nose up toward the hairline; then, placing your fingers over the eyebrows, work up toward the hairline; finally, place your fingertips in the center of the forehead and work out toward the temples.

Try these other types of facial massage as well. These different massage techniques may be used singly or combined for a marvelously refreshing experience.

Finger circles

Following the same instructions, make smaller circular movements with your fingers, pressing, then releasing pressure as you very gradually move toward the ear. As you massage through the different areas of the face, don't lift or move the fingers over the surface of the skin. Instead, try to create pressure that will go through to the muscle below the skin.

Patting

With the tips of the three middle fingers, tap the skin quickly and gently, flapping your hand up and down from the wrist. Don't drag the skin; simply tap it, moving speedily through the different facial massage areas.

Back massage

Place your hands palms down on the lower back, thumbs together and fingers pointing out toward the sides. Place your palms gently so that the thumbs and fingertips fit the depressions between the muscles while the palm covers the muscle. Exerting pressure, stroke upward toward the armpits. Next, follow the line of the spine, working up toward the neck, stroking on either side of the spine. The pressure should be continuous and as deep as is comfortable. Stroke back to the starting position and again gradually work over the entire back.

Repeat the entire procedure but this time use the rolling technique.

After *stroking* and *rolling*, place your palms in the starting position on the back and knead the muscles throughout the back. Knead up and down from side to side. Next, knead along the sides of the waist.

eating for fitness

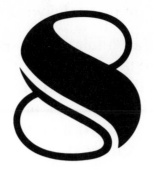

A s EVERYONE is aware these days, good nutrition is as important in keeping fit as exercise is. Learning to eat healthfully can be a positive and exciting experience and, like exercise, it helps to do it with a friend.

In this chapter I'm going to outline the basic dos and don'ts of eating to keep fit. I'm also including a three-day menu plan that you can use as a guide. Further suggested reading on diet and nutrition appears on pages 209–210.

What to eat

Your basic rules should be "Everything in moderation" and "Fresh is best." Try to eat as much fresh unprocessed food as possible. Fresh food is not only higher in nutritional value, it tastes better, too! If you buy processed foods, be sure to read the label first. Many products have high sugar and salt contents. Sugar is often disguised as corn syrup, dextrose, maltose, or glucose. Once you get into the habit of reading labels, you'll be amazed at how often the products they describe contain more sugar, salt, and sheer chemicals than anything else. Unless it is terribly impractical, try to do without processed food as much as you can. I generally keep them out of my kitchen altogether.

The chart, "New American Eating Guide," from the Center for Science in the Public Interest (see pages 214–215) shows not only the four food groups but also their recommended daily portions.

It's important to restrict your intake of foods we know contribute to ill health. The main culprits are fats, refined sugar, salt, and caffeine. It's not realistic to believe that you can go through life without ever indulging in any of these things again, but you can learn to be selective. Unless you have orders to the contrary from your doctor, I believe that you can eat everything. Just don't go to extremes!

FATS: Learn to substitute low-fat foods for high-fat ones. Look for dairy products that contain skim instead of whole milk. If you dislike the taste of skim milk, do what I do: mix it with whole milk so that it's only half skim. Or buy 2-percent milk, which amounts to about the same thing (whole milk is 4 percent butterfat).

Yogurt is another product that works well as a substitute. Plain low-fat yogurt can be used in almost any recipe calling for sour cream or even heavy cream. Most of the time you can't tell, and when you can it usually tastes better! Plain yogurt also tastes wonderful as a dressing for steamed fresh vegetables, and mixed with strawberries or other fruits it makes a delicious dessert.

SUGAR AND SALT: Scientific studies have demonstrated that too much refined sugar contributes to obesity, heart disease, diabetes, and many other illnesses. Moreover, a constant onslaught of sugar on the teeth creates an atmosphere where only decay can be the winner. It's a good idea to rinse your mouth out with water every time you have something sugary, so that at least some of the harmful sticky residue is washed away. Sugar's biggest fault is that it contains calories with no nutritional value. Sugar cheats the body out of the vitamins and minerals it needs for optimum health. Try to use honey as a sweetener instead. Ounce for ounce it's sweeter than white sugar so not only will less honey yield the desired sweetness, but it also contains some copper, iron, calcium, potassium, plus smaller quantities of additional minerals and *all* of the eight essential amino acids.

Too much salt causes high blood pressure and water retention. It can also interfere with the body's ability to absorb vitamins and minerals. While your body needs *some* salt, in large doses salt acts like a poison. When the kidneys can't handle an excess supply of it, your body stores it in your lower extremities, your legs. Concurrently, your body takes measures to protect itself from the toxic effects of the salt by bringing water to the same areas where the salt is being held to dilute it. The resulting edema, or swelling, causes discomfort and worse.

Try to salt sparingly, if at all. Before you do salt, taste your food. It just may not need any!

CAFFEINE: The truth is that caffeine is a drug, and one that most of us are addicted to very early on. I grew up in a home where the coffee pot was always hot and at a moment's notice someone would pour a cup and sit down to talk. Before I weaned myself from coffee, I was consuming up to ten cups a day! Now my limit is two cups daily. Coffee is not the only caffeine-laden drink around, though it does seem to be the most popular. Tea, cocoa, chocolate, and many soft drinks also contain caffeine.

Too much caffeine may be instrumental in producing abnormal heart rhythms, rapid heartbeat, and sometimes an extra heartbeat. It can make you nervous, anxious, and jittery. There is evidence that caffeine contributes to digestive disorders such as heartburn and upset stomach and can increase the risk of bladder cancer. Since there is also some evidence that caffeine causes birth defects, no pregnant woman should consume more than two cups a day, and that much only with her doctor's approval.

The best way to break yourself of the caffeine habit is to do it gradually. Because it is addictive both psychologically and physically, caffeine withdrawal is a major problem. An abrupt withdrawal can cause such symptoms as headache, nervousness, depression, and drowsiness. Reduce your intake a little every day until you are consuming no more than two cups, or even none at all.

There are many alternatives to caffeine. There's decaffeinated coffee as well as a large selection of herbal teas. Try carob instead of chocolate. Rather than reaching for a soft drink, try fruit juice or juice combined with seltzer or sparkling mineral water. Not as accessible, but certainly available are satisfying grain-based beverages made from bran, wheat, molasses, or barley.

ALCOHOL: Moderation applies here, too. It's also a good idea to eat before you drink. Choose something high in protein, starch, or fat: peanut butter or cheese and crackers, or a glass of whole milk. This coats your stomach and slows down alcohol absorption. Avoid salty snack foods—they make you thirsty and so increase the chance that you'll drink too much. At the end of a hard, tense, and nervous day, a drink sipped (not gulped!) can help you wind down. But if you take more than that, you may be asking for trouble. So, please, drink intelligently!

Some words of caution if you are pregnant: *Don't drink.* Alcohol is harmful to both mother and fetus. For both your sakes, drink juice or water.

VITAMINS: One thing the experts definitely don't agree on is whether we need to take vitamins at all. Some insist that if you eat properly you'll get all the vitamins you need and that taking vitamin supplements is foolish, expensive, and sometimes even harmful. Whereas I agree with these arguments in theory, in practice I favor the experts who encourage taking vitamin supplements. I think they're necessary because it's quite possible, even probable, that we do not receive the full vitamin potential from the foods we eat. Cattle and poultry are pumped full of antibiotics and other chemicals; fish have to survive in increasingly polluted waters. Fruits and vegetables are dusted with toxic insecticides, and the crops themselves are picked and shipped while they are still green. And on and on.

So I favor taking a multivitamin and mineral supplement daily, just to be on the safe side. If you feel it is necessary, an additional "high-stress" B vitamin plus vitamins C and E would be good. If you feel unsure of your vitamin needs, ask your doctor to perform special tests to measure the level of vitamins and minerals in your system.

How to eat out: Parties and restaurants

Although party hosts and restaurateurs are increasingly sensitive to the growing health orientation of their guests, it is still best to create your own "health action plan" before you go anywhere.

If you're going to a cocktail party, eat a little something beforehand so you won't be tempted by the more fattening and less nutritious party food (unless your host is a health buff too and has laid out a spread of crudités and other healthy goodies!) The same rule applies to dinner parties, unless you know your hosts have the same food orientation as you do. Then you can eat only a little of everything. It is not necessary to make a point of refusing a particularly rich or calorie-laden dish.

In a restaurant, the real problem is often the sauce or dressing. Ask to have your dish without it or with it on the side. As for that tempting and very gloppy dessert, pass it by. These days most restaurants offer fresh fruits in addition to pastries. Indulge in the fresh raspberries, not the raspberry tart!

Establishing the good-eating habit

When people decide to change their eating habits, they often go to extremes and eliminate everything even vaguely unhealthy. Inevitably, this includes all their favorite treats! The only thing this accomplishes is to make the treats take on greater importance. If you love ice cream or chocolate or anything falling into the not-so-healthy or even the junk category, allow yourself to indulge from time to time. If you're usually selective about your food and on the whole opt for a healthy life-style, an occasional indiscretion won't hurt you. In fact, the pleasure derived will do a lot to boost your spirits and will help to keep those treats from turning into obsessions—and thereby wrecking your health-oriented food program.

Try to have a clear understanding of the true meaning of food in your life. We have all sorts of reasons for eating—most of them poor ones. Food will not cure loneliness nor make us feel loved. As more studies are done about various kinds of food and our reactions to them, however, we are learning that certain foods can have a tremendous effect on some people, both physically and mentally. Keep track of any reaction you have to different foods. If you find that you suffer extreme mood swings or depressions, do yourself a favor and have your doctor do some tests. You might have a mild allergy; wheat, milk, eggs, and seafood are the most common culprits. (If you are strongly allergic, you've probably known it for some time.) Many illnesses have been discovered to originate in the diet, and diabetes, hypoglycemia, and gastrointestinal disorders can often be traced to a specific food. Obviously, if the wrong diet can make you sick, then a proper diet can make you well.

Listen to your body! The main purpose of food is to give your body the fuel it needs to stay healthy and the material it needs to build and repair tissues and organs. It should supply the vitamins, minerals, and nutrients to give you clear skin, sturdy bones, and shining hair. But you must make the right choices to give your body the energy it needs.

Almost as important as *what* you eat is *how* you eat. Make each meal an occasion. Think about what you feel like eating and pick those foods that will do the most for your body. Take the time to chew properly and appreciate the taste of your meal. If you munch away in a nervous hurry, your food will be digested inefficiently. If you learn to eat slowly, not only will you enjoy your food more, but you'll find you tend to eat less. It's better to postpone a meal than to eat it in a hurry. You might even consider having several small meals spread out over the course of a day, rather than one or two heavy meals.

The plan

Here's a three-day menu plan that combines foods that are not only crammed full of vitamins and minerals for good health but also loaded with the fuel you need for an abundance of energy. These menus are just suggestions. I'm sure you'll want to try your hand at putting together healthy, well-balanced meals geared toward your own tastes. I've found that my body usually makes its needs quite clear to me and I'm always aware of what foods are necessary at each meal.

Although the meals in this menu plan will most likely be prepared at home, I've tried to choose foods that would also be available in a restaurant or lend themselves to a "brown bag special" to be eaten at your desk. Just remember, be creative and choose healthy foods that you like. Eat until you're pleasantly full but never stuffed.

Try these hints for healthy eating:

Eat a high-energy breakfast.

Try to eat your largest meal early in the day. Your evening meal should be as light and as early as possible.

If you must snack before bed, good choices are fruit or yogurt or a glass of milk. Foods high in calcium are always a good choice for an evening snack, and dairy products contain the amino acid tryptophan, which works as a natural tranquilizer.

Drink lots of liquids, preferably water, during the day. Six to eight glasses is not too much.

It's really best to go to bed slightly hungry. If your digestive system is working hard all night, you won't be able to get the refreshing, restful sleep you need.

DAY ONE

Breakfast
1 slice whole wheat toast
1 oz. hard cheese or 1 egg (poached or boiled)
fresh fruit with 1 c. yogurt
coffee or tea

Lunch
6 oz. tomato juice
chicken, tuna, turkey, or seafood salad; dressing on the side
melon
tea or herb beverage

Dinner
roast chicken or meat loaf
Brussels sprouts
brown rice
tea or herb beverage

Snack
1 orange

DAY TWO

Breakfast
6 oz. orange juice
oatmeal with 4 oz. milk and a sprinkling of raisins
1 slice whole wheat toast
coffee or tea

Lunch
pasta with vegetables (Spaghetti Primavera, for instance)
green salad with lemon juice
melon or berries with or without yogurt

Dinner
broiled fish
steamed broccoli with 1 T. yogurt as a sauce
baked potato
1 glass skim milk

Snack
1 banana or apple

DAY THREE

Breakfast

half grapefruit
1 slice whole wheat toast spread with
    1 T. peanut butter
1 banana
1 glass skim milk
coffee or tea

Lunch

lentil soup
Caesar salad
crusty bread

fresh fruit salad (with yogurt if desired)
tea or herb beverage

Dinner

1 slice whole wheat toast
mushroom and chicken liver omelet
steamed zucchini
tea or herb beverage

Snack

1 c. plain yogurt sprinkled with wheat
    germ and 1 t. honey, if desired

keeping it all together

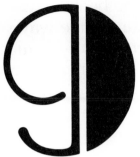

*I*F YOU'VE JUST finished reading this book but have not yet embarked on the exercises, I hope you're eager to start. If you're that lucky couple who are just completing the eight-week fitness program, I know that you both feel and look wonderful and have more energy than ever before! I'll wager that your sex life has improved as well and that you are experiencing a kind of closeness and intimacy with your partner that you've never known before.

Well, now's the time to take advantage of this high to expand into other areas of fitness. Since you enjoy being physical together, why not try sharing some sports too? How about tennis or racketball? Jogging in the morning or swimming some laps together at the end of the day or both? The possibilities are limitless. Just use your imaginations and you can find ways not only to expand your fitness regimen, but to create additional time to spend together.

Now that you've gotten to the top of your fitness form, are you concerned that you might not be able to keep it all together? Well, have no fear. Being slim, trim, feeling and looking great is frequently incentive enough to keep you from backsliding. Don't be concerned if you slip occasionally. We all do. But don't let a small slip become an excuse for further decline. Get yourself right back on program! It shouldn't be hard now that you have an ally—someone you can turn to for encouragement and support. Both of you should continue working together on the fitness program a minimum of once a week. If you can do it more often, all the better! Continuing on the program three times a week can only enhance your lives by making you even healthier and more fit.

Most of all, take pleasure in the way you look and feel now. And don't forget to let each other know how much you love the way his or her slim, trim, healthy body looks (in or out of clothes!). The glow of good health is something to take considerable pride in. You have been good to yourselves in the best possible way human beings can be!

suggested reading

For further instruction on how to unwind while getting close to that special person through massage, here are two of the most useful books I have found on the subject:

Downing, George. *The Massage Book*. New York: Random House/ Bookworks, 1972.

This is the most complete and easy to understand introduction to all the different kinds of massage. It is profusely illustrated, showing step-by-step hand positions, hand motions, and how to apply your technique to different areas of the body.

Meagher, Jack, and Boughton, Pat. *Sports-Massage*. New York: Doubleday/Dolphin, 1980.

This is just what the title says: massage to prepare your body for specific sports— for instance, special arm and shoulder massages for tennis players.

There are hundreds of relaxation techniques and just as many books about them. Here are a few of my favorites:

Forem, Jack. *Transcendental Meditation*. New York: E. P. Dutton, 1974.

This is one of the best known books about TM and how the TM movement started. It covers the complex psychology behind the simple technique that became one of America's foremost relaxation and meditation methods.

Benson, Herbert, M.D. *The Relaxation Response*. New York: Avon Books, 1976.

This book is a classic: a simple, easy-to-understand guide for reducing stress and tension.

Stroebel, Charles F., M.D. *QR: The Quieting Reflex*. New York: G. P. Putnam's, 1982.

A renowned medical expert on stress and stress management explains the basic steps and exercises for mastering a six-second technique for coping with stress anytime, anywhere. Once learned, the technique becomes automatic.

Hittleman, Richard. *Guide to Yoga Meditation*. New York: Bantam Books, 1981.

This one is a classic, a revision of the 1969 book. Richard Hittleman was one of the first people, back in the mid-sixties, to make yoga a household word. Through his many books (all of which are good and informative) and his television show, he translated the ancient techniques of yoga into a language the American public could understand. In my opinion, he's chiefly responsible for introducing yoga, with all its positive influences, to literally millions of people. This book is a basic primer and an excellent starting point for anyone interested in yoga.

Knowing yourself and your needs is an important first step toward building intimacy with others. I think you will find the following books very helpful:

Montagu, Ashley. *Touching: The Human Significance of the Skin*, 2nd ed. New York: Harper & Row, 1978.
In this inspiring book, anthropologist Montagu gives us the scientific answers to why touching is so pleasurable, both on a physical and psychological level, and, indeed, why it is necessary for the existence of life itself.

Fast, Julius. *Body Language*. New York: Pocket Books, 1975.
A basic guide to make you aware of how you respond to your partner and vice versa.

The following books are written by medical doctors, and help to explain, in layman's language, what stress is, what medicine has learned about it, and how you can try to control it.

Selye, Hans, M.D. *The Stress of Life*, rev. ed. New York: McGraw-Hill, 1976.

A very famous book and still one of the best! It is medically oriented, but explains in simple terms how to convert stress into positive energy.

DeRosis, Helen, M.D. *Women and Anxiety*. New York: Delacorte Press, 1979.
An important book for both men and women. It deals with the effect of stress on women's hormones, something all couples should be aware of, since certain stresses can affect women very differently than they do men.

Samuels, Mike, M.D., and Bennett, Hal. *The Well Body Book*. New York: Random House/Bookworks, 1973.
Here's a total self-care book, giving you information about everything you need to know to keep your body well. Among the topics: massage, relaxation, how different organs of the body function, proper nutrition, simple home remedies, and how to diagnose yourself. It doesn't replace a doctor, nor does it intend to, but it does give you a lot of sound basic medical advice.

There are literally hundreds of worthwhile nutrition and diet books available. Since choosing can be a problem, here are a few of my favorites. They are crammed full of information about nutrition, diet, and vitamins. I enjoyed and strongly recommend them.

Brody, Jane. *Jane Brody's Nutrition Book*. New York: W. W. Norton, 1981.
This book is a must for people who are serious about what and how they eat.

Gross, Joy. *The 30-Day Way to a Born-Again Body.* New York: Berkley, 1981.

I've had the pleasure of meeting Joy and, without a doubt, she's a beautiful and healthy example of just how successful her approach toward nutrition, health, and exercise is.

Fredericks, Carlton. *Food Facts & Fallacies.* New York: Arc Books, 1971.

Carlton Fredericks has written many nutrition books. I think this is one of his best.

Want a better understanding of *why* you have specific weight problems? Do you have a desire to reeducate yourself and improve your eating habits? The following books could help:

Linn, Robert. *Staying Thin.* New York: G. P. Putnam's, 1980.

Dr. Linn is one of the top nutritional authorities in the country. I feel lucky to have worked with him on a number of occasions. He's written several books, but this is one I particularly enjoyed. It's full of positive and constructive advice about how to get thin and, most important, how to *stay* thin.

Edelstein, Barbara. *The Woman Doctor's Diet for Women.* Englewood Cliffs, N.J.: Prentice Hall, 1977.

A no-frills, no-nonsense diet book for people (both men and women) who want to take weight off and keep it off!

Myerson, Bess, and Adler, Bill. *The I Love N.Y. Diet.* New York: William Morrow, 1982.

This diet is based on one originally developed by the Bureau of Nutrition, New York City Department of Health. It's safe, sensible, and it really works.

Pritikin, Nathan. *The Pritikin Program for Diet & Exercise.* New York: Bantam, 1980.

Many millions have lost weight and improved their health by following this fine program.

In my opinion anything written by Adelle Davis is worth reading. Adelle Davis was one of the pioneers of modern nutrition, way back in the fifties. These books are classics, and they are still bought by the millions each year by people who are interested in eating properly and who want good, concrete nutritional advice.

Davis, Adelle. *Let's Eat Right and Keep Fit.* New York: New American Library, 1970.

————. *Let's Get Well.* New York: New American Library, 1972.

————. *Let's Cook It Right.* New York: New American Library, 1970.

I'd like to mention two other books without which in my kitchen I'd be lost. After all, it's quite clear that you must know how to prepare and serve healthy, delicious meals if you're sincere about how you look and feel:

Ewald, Ellen Buchman. *Recipes for a Small Planet,* New York: Ballantine, 1982.

If you want a book that takes all the guesswork out of dieting here's a terrific one:

Weight Watchers 365-Day Menu Cookbook. New York: New American Library, 1982.

THE PROGRAM

WEEKS	DAY 1 Exercise Group	Group Total	DAY 2 Exercise Group	Group Total	DAY 3 Exercise Group	Group Total
1 and 2 choose from the easy section (E)	A—Warm-up B C D F—Cool-down	10 3 4 3 10	A—Warm-up B C D E1—Cardiovascular F—Cool-down	10 3 3 4 10	A—Warm-up B C D F—Cool-down	10 4 3 3 10
3 and 4 choose from the medium section (M)	A—Warm-up B C D F—Cool-down	10 4 7 4 10	A—Warm-up B C D E1 or E2—Cardiovascular F—Cool-down	10 3 3 4 10	A—Warm-up B C D F—Cool-down	10 7 4 4 10
5 and 6 choose from the hard section (H)	A—Warm-up B C D F—Cool-down	10 4 7 4 10	A—Warm-up B C D E2—Cardiovascular F—Cool-down	10 3 3 4 10	A—Warm-up B C D F—Cool-down	10 7 4 4 10
7 and 8 choose from the hard section (wrist and ankle weights optional) (H)	A—Warm-up B C D F—Cool-down	10 4 7 4 10	A—Warm-up B C D E3—Cardiovascular F—Cool-down	10 3 3 4 10	A—Warm-up B C D F—Cool-down	10 7 4 4 10

SAMPLE EXERCISE PROGRAM

WEEKS		DAY 1			DAY 2			DAY 3	
	Exercise Group	Group Total	Exercise Name	Exercise Group	Group Total	Exercise Name	Exercise Group	Group Total	Exercise Name
1 and 2 EASY (E)	A	10	Warm-up—do all	A	10	Warm-up—do all	A	10	Warm-up—do all
	B	3	Pendulum Lift Follow-up	B	3	Inward-Outward Press Triangle Forward Hold	B	4	Backward Push-up Shrug Crisscross Pendulum
	C	4	Spring Forward-Back Circle Foot Push	C	3	Foot Push Fold Big Push	C	3	Circle Easy Up Leg-out
	D	3	Ankle Spread Knee Press Bicycle	D	4	Rolling Knee Press High Hip Press Crossover Bicycle	D	3	Elevator Under the Bridge Stroll
				E1	10	Cardiovascular			
	F	10	Cool-down—do all	F	10	Cool-down—do all	F	10	Cool-down—do all
3 and 4 MEDIUM (M)	A	10	Warm-up—do all	A	10	Warm-up—do all	A	10	Warm-up—do all
	B	4	Windmill Bear Hug Locomotion Inward-Outward Press Too	B	3	Airplane Roundabout Brick Wall	B	7	Up Lift Push-out Together Cobra Windmill Inward-Outward Press Too Airplane Roundabout
	C	7	Release Back Fold Too Bookends Star Lift Piggyback Leg-go-round Climbing Foot Push	C	3	Star Lift Tilt Piggyback	C	4	Climbing Foot Push Lean Back Leg-go-round Bigger Push
				D	4	Together Split High Kicker Stroll Too Hip Push			

5 and 6 / 7 and 8

Exercise Group	Group Total	Exercise Name
D	4	Leg Lift with Resistance / Hip Push / High Kicker / Together Split
F	10	Cool-down—do all

E1 or E2*

Exercise Group	Group Total	Exercise Name
A	10	Warm-up—do all
B	3	Together Lift / Bottoms Up / Come Hither
C	3	A Bicycle Built for Two / Fold-over / Curl-up Together
D	4	Twisting T / Thigh Lift Too / Hike / Sideways Pull
E2 or E3*		Cardiovascular
F	10	Cool-down—do all

Exercise Group	Group Total	Exercise Name
A	10	Warm-up—do all
B	7	Butterfly / Pump / Together Again Cobra / Come Hither / Tug / Bottoms Up / Back Lift
C	4	Circle Too / Side Back Twist / Blossom / Star Lift Too
D	4	Toe-Down Lift / Swan / Hip Lift with Friend / Hike
F	10	Cool-down—do all

	Group Total	Exercise Name
D	4	Bridge / Stroll Too / Thigh Lift / Swinging Palm
F	10	Cool-down—do all

HARD 〔H〕

Exercise Group	Group Total	Exercise Name
A	10	Warm-up—do all
B	4	Back Lift / Tug / Accordion / Pyramid Lift
C	7	Blossom / Curl-up Together / Fold-over / Star Lift Too / A Bicycle Built for Two / Circle Too / Side Back Twist
D	4	Twisting T / Split Lift / Sideways Pull / Toe-Down Lift
F	10	Cool-down—do all

*Whichever cardiovascular series you've progressed to.

213

NEW AMERICAN EATING GUIDE*

	ANYTIME	IN MODERATION	NOW AND THEN
Group 1 Beans, Grains, and Nuts four or more servings a day	bread and rolls (whole grain) bulghur dried beans and peas (legumes) lentils oatmeal pasta, whole wheat rice, brown rye bread sprouts whole grain hot and cold cereal whole wheat matzoh	cornbread **8** flour tortilla **8** hominy grits **8** macaroni and cheese **1**,**(6)**,**8** matzoh **8** nuts **3** pasta, except whole wheat **8** peanut butter **3** pizza **6**,**8** refined, unsweetened cereals **8** refried beans, commercial **1**, homemade in oil **2** seeds **3** soybeans **2** tofu **2** waffles or pancakes, syrup **5**,**(6)**,**8** white bread and rolls **8** white rice **8**	croissant **4**,**8** doughnut (yeast leavened) **3 or 4**,**5**,**8** presweetened breakfast cereals **5**,**8** sticky buns **1 or 2**,**5**,**8** stuffing, made with butter **4**,**(6)**,**8**
Group 2 Fruits and Vegetables four or more servings a day	all fruits and vegetables except those listed at right applesauce (unsweetened) unsweetened fruit juices unsalted vegetable juices potatoes, white or sweet	avocado **3** cole slaw **3** cranberry sauce (canned) **5** dried fruit french fries, homemade in vegetable oil **2**, commercial **1** fried eggplant (veg. oil) **2** fruits canned in syrup **5** gazpacho **2**,**(6)** glazed carrots **5**,**(6)** guacamole **3** potatoes au gratin **1**,**(6)** salted vegetable juices **6** sweetened fruit juices **5** vegetables canned with salt **6**	coconut **4** pickles **6**

214

Group 3 Milk Products two servings a day	buttermilk made from skim milk lassi (low-fat yogurt and fruit juice drink) low-fat cottage cheese low-fat milk, 1% milkfat low-fat yogurt nonfat dry milk skim milk cheeses **(6)** skim milk skim milk and banana shake	cocoa made with skim milk **5** cottage cheese, regular, 4% milkfat **1** frozen low-fat yogurt **5** ice milk **5** low-fat milk, 2% milkfat **1** low-fat yogurt, sweetened **5** mozzarella cheese, part-skim type only **1,(6)**	cheesecake **4,5** cheese fondue **4,(6)** cheese soufflé **4,(6),7** eggnog **1,5,7** hard cheeses: blue, brick, Camembert, cheddar, Muenster, Swiss **4,(6)** ice cream **4,5** processed cheeses **4,6** whole milk **4** whole milk yogurt **4**
Group 4 Poultry, Fish, Meat, and Eggs two servings a day Vegetarians: nutrients in these foods can be obtained by eating more foods in groups 1, 2, and 3	FISH cod flounder gefilte fish **(6)** haddock halibut perch pollack rockfish shellfish, except shrimp sole tuna, water packed **(6)** EGG PRODUCTS egg whites only POULTRY chicken or turkey, boiled, baked, or roasted (no skin)	FISH (drained well if canned) fried fish **1 or 2** herring **3,6** mackerel, canned **2,(6)** salmon, pink, canned **2,(6)** sardines **2,(6)** shrimp **7** tuna, oil-packed **2,(6)** POULTRY chicken liver, baked or broiled, **7** (just one!) fried chicken, homemade in vegetable oil **3** chicken or turkey, boiled, baked or roasted (with skin) **2** RED MEATS (trimmed of all outside fat!) flank steak **1** leg or loin of lamb **1** pork shoulder or loin, lean **1** round steak or ground round **1** rump roast **1** sirloin steak, lean **1** veal **1**	POULTRY fried chicken, commercially prepared **4** EGG cheese omelet **4,7** egg yolk or whole egg (about 3 per week) **3,7** RED MEATS bacon **4,(6)** beef liver, fried **1,7** bologna **4,6** corned beef **4,6** ground beef **4** ham, trimmed well **1,6** hot dogs **4,6** liverwurst **4,6** pig's feet **4** salami **4,6** sausage **4,6** spare ribs **4** untrimmed red meats **4**

KEY: **1**-moderate fat, saturated **2**-moderate fat, unsaturated **3**-high fat, saturated **4**-high fat, saturated **5**-high in added sugar **6**-high in salt or sodium **(6)**-may be high in salt or sodium **7**-high in cholesterol **8**-refined grains

*Reprinted from New American Eating Guide which is available from the Center for Science in the Public Interest, 1755 S Street, N.W., Washington, D.C., 20009, for $3.00, $6.00 laminated, copyright 1979.

ABOUT THE AUTHOR

Carol Gregor is a recognized authority in the field of physical fitness. Ms. Gregor currently serves as consultant to *Woman's Day, The Sophisticate's Beauty Guide* and *Sophisticate's Hair Guide.* She regularly contributes articles and devises exercises for publications such as *Good Housekeeping, Family Circle, Vogue, Cosmopolitan, Mademoiselle, Harper's Bazaar, Women's Wear Daily* and *W.* In addition, Carol and her exercise technique, "Body Awareness," have been featured in *Working Woman, New York Daily News, The New York Times, New York Post* and eighteen of the newspapers in the Gannett chain.

Teaching has remained an integral part of Ms. Gregor's professional schedule. For fifteen years she has directed the Body Awareness Program. For a number of these years her program was at Bergdorf Goodman in New York City. Today, in addition to teaching her select private clientele and classes, she is frequently invited by corporations to work with employee groups.

Ms. Gregor lives in New York City.